Exam-Oriented OBSTETRICS and GYNAECOLOGY

QUESTIONS and ANSWERS

Exam-Oriented OBSTETRICS and GYNAECOLOGY

QUESTIONS and ANSWERS

K. Mukhopadhyay
MD, FCGP, PGCCHFWM

Associate Professor
College of Medicine and JNM Hospital
Kalyani, West Bengal

CBS

CBS Publishers & Distributors Pvt. Ltd.

New Delhi • Bengaluru • Chennai • Kochi • Kolkata • Mumbai
Hyderabad • Nagpur • Patna • Pune • Vijayawada

ISBN: 978-81-239-1929-4

First Edition: 2011
Reprint: 2012, 2017

Published by **Satish Kumar Jain** and produced by **Varun Jain** for
CBS Publishers & Distributors Pvt. Ltd.,
4819/XI Prahlad Street, 24 Ansari Road, Daryaganj, New Delhi - 110002
delhi@cbspd.com, cbspubs@airtelmail.in • www.cbspd.com
Ph.: 23289259, 23266861, 23266867 • Fax: 011-23243014

Corporate Office: 204 FIE, Industrial Area, Patparganj, Delhi - 110 092
Ph: 49344934 • Fax: 011-49344935
E-mail: publishing@cbspd.com • publicity@cbspd.com

Branches:
- ***Bengaluru:*** 2975, 17th Cross, K.R. Road, Bansankari 2nd Stage, Bengaluru - 70 • Ph: +91-80-26771678/79 • Fax: +91-80-26771680 E-mail: cbsbng@gmail.com, bangalore@cbspd.com
- ***Chennai:*** No. 7, Subbaraya Street, Shenoy Nagar, Chennai - 600030 Ph: +91-44-26681266, 26680620 • Fax: +91-44-42032115 E-mail: chennai@cbspd.com
- ***Kochi:*** Ashana House, 39/1904, A.M. Thomas Road, Valanjambalam, Ernakulum, Kochi • Ph: +91-484-4059061-65 Fax: +91-484-4059065 • E-mail: cochin@cbspd.com
- ***Kolkata:*** 6-B, Ground Floor, Rameshwar Shaw Road, Kolkata - 700014 Ph: +91-33-22891126/7/8 • E-mail: kolkata@cbspd.com
- ***Mumbai:*** 83-C, Dr. E. Moses Road, Worli, Mumbai - 400018 Ph: +91-9833017933, 022-24902340/41 • E-mail: mumbai@cbspd.com

Representatives:
- Hyderabad: 0-9885175004
- Patna: 0-9334159340
- Vijayawada: 0-9000660880
- Nagpur: 0-9021734563
- Pune: 0-9623451994

Printed at:
India Binding House, Noida, UP (India)

Preface

Nothing is more exciting than private general practice where knowledge of every discipline of medical science is important. I bestow this book **Exam-Oriented Obstetrics and Gynaecology** to the general practitioners and undergraduate medical students in QUESTION and ANSWER format. Any suggestions from students, teachers and practitioners are welcome.

At this juncture I remember my teachers Prof PK Chaudhary, Prof A Chakraverty, Prof TN Mukherjee, Prof P Dasgupta, Prof B Mondal and Dr Banoshree Ghosh whose lectures were of tremendous help in preparing this book.

Dr Ashim Biswas, Dr Manjit Singh Sindhu, Dr Manidip Paul, Dr MM Kolay, Dr J Mukherjee, Dr A Mukhopadhyay, Dr (Mrs) S Mukhopadhyay, Dr (Mrs) B. Mukherjee, Mr S Chatterjee, Mr Basudeb Mukherjee, Mr Baladeb Mukherjee, Mrs Jayanti Sinha, Mr Anil Kumar Singh, Mrs Lakshmi Chatterjee, Mrs Aditi Banerjee, Mrs Arundhati Banerjee, Mrs Nandini Pandit, Miss Anuradha Sinha, Mr Mrinal Sinha, Mr Alok Kumar Pal, Mr and Mrs TK Lahiri, Prof D Das and Prof A Banerjee of MGM Medical College, Kishanganj, encouraged me to write this book.

Dr (Mrs) Barnali Mukherjee has helped me by drawing some of the important illustrations in this book.

My mother Mrs Baid Bani Mukherjee went through infinite patience and always stood by me.

I thank Mr SK Jain, Managing Director, and Mr YN Arjuna, Publishing Director, of CBS Publishers & Distributors, New Delhi, for bringing out this book.

Mr Ramanand Kr. Singh of M/s Singh Graphics, Dhanbad, helped me in preparing the typescript of this book, my sincere thanks to him.

K. Mukhopadhay

to

Late Satadal Basani Devi

Late Bina Mukherjee

Smt Baid Bani Mukherjee

Smt Kajoli Mukherjee

Contents

Section 2
Neonate Care

Section 3
Gynaecology

Section 1
Obstetrics

- Anatomy and Physiology of Female Genital Organs
- Diagnosis of Pregnancy
- Antenatal Care
- Haemorrhage in Early Pregnancy
- Ectopic Pregnancy
- Antepartum Haemorrhage
- Toxaemias of Pregnacy
- Some Diseases in Pregnacny
- Diseases of Genital Tract in Pregnancy
- Preterm Labour; Post-term Pregnancy
- Normal Labour
- Complications of Third Stage Labour
- Abnormal Presentation
- Multiple Pregnancy: Hydramnios
- Abnormal Umbilical Cord and Foetal Anomalies
- Cephalopelvic Disproportion
- Abnormal Uterine Contraction
- Maternal Injuries in Labour
- Puerperium
- Operations in Obstetrics
- Drugs Acting on Uterus

Anatomy and Physiology of Female Genital Organs

1

LAQ 1 How the following organs are developed.
(1) Uterus and fallopian tube (2) Vagina (3) Female genitalia.

Uterus and Fallopian Tube

The epithelium of uterus develops from fused paramesonephric duct. The myometrium develops from surrounding mesoderm. Uterine tube or fallopian tube develops from proximal vertical parts of paramesonephric duct. The intermediate horizontal parts produce fundus and body of uterus. The caudal vertical part fuse with each other, and median portion disappears to produce lower parts of body of uterus and cervix of uterus.

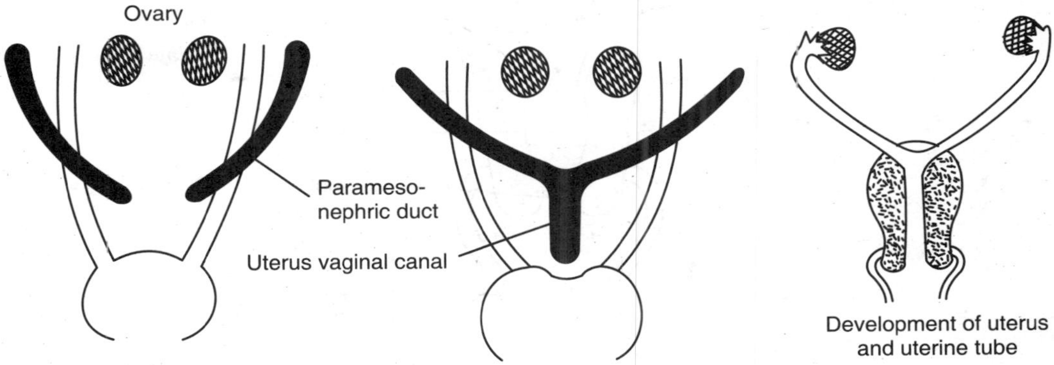

Development of uterus and uterine tube

Vagina

The fused uterovaginal canal comes in contact with dorsal wall of urogenital sinus. Urogenital sinus and uterovaginal canal are separated by formation of solid plate of cells called vaginal canal.

Endodermal cells of urogenital sinus proliferate to form two swelling called sinovaginal bulbs which fuse to form vaginal plate, a lumen is formed in vaginal plate, which produces vagina.

Female Genitalia

Cloacal membrane subdivided into ventral urogenital membrane and dorsal anal membrane by urorectal septum. Urogenital membrane elongates craniocaudally and three elevations of mesoderm appear by the side of it, called genital tubercle and right and left genital swelling. The genital tubercle produces clitoris and genital swelling enlarges to form labia majora which fuses posteriorly to produce posterior commissure.

SAQ 2 What are the parts of vulva or external genitalia?

(i) Mons pubis, (ii) labia majora, (iii) labia minora, (iv) clitoris, (v) vestibule with: (a) external urethral opening, (b) vaginal orifice and hymen, (c) ducts of Bartholin gland.

LAQ 3 Describe the anatomy of uterus.

Uterus is pelvic organ behind bladder and rectum in front. Fallopian tube opens in its superolateral angle, opens into vagina by external os. Weighing 30–40 gm. Its length, breadth, thickness are 3:2:1 inches, respectively. It consists of fundus, body and cervix. The angle between body and cervix is 120–125° (anteflexed) and angle of long axis of uterus and vagina is about 90° (called anteversion). In anterior surface, peritoneum reflects up to isthmus (junction of body and cervix of uterus) producing uterovesical pouch. On posterior wall, peritoneum reflects up to vagina and middle and lower one-third of rectum producing pouch of Douglas.

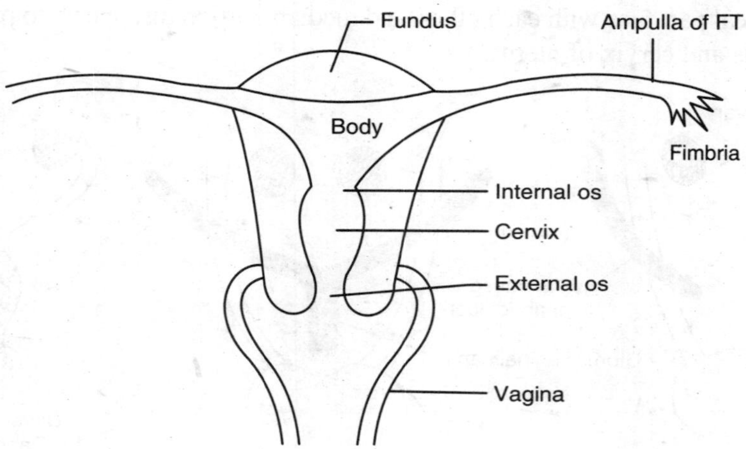

Ligaments and supports of uterus

True non-peritoneal ligaments

(i) Round ligament.
(ii) Uterosacral ligament.
(iii) Pubocervical ligament.
(iv) Mackenrodt's ligament.

False peritoneal ligaments

(i) Uterovesical fold (anterior ligament)
(ii) Rectovaginal fold (posterior ligament)
(iii) Broad ligaments 2 in numbers.

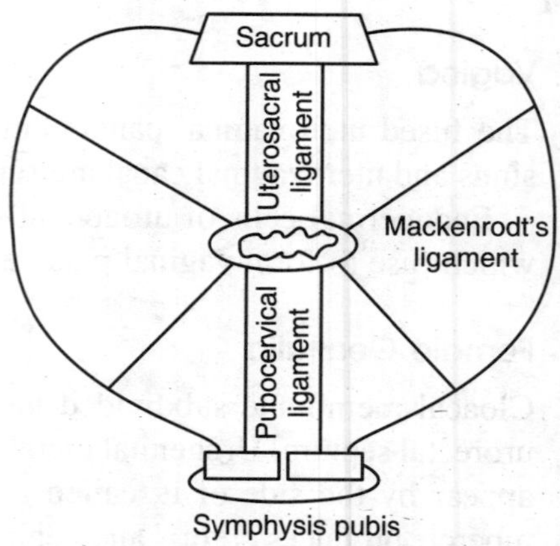

Ligaments of uterus

Arterial supply: (i) Uterine artery—a branch of anterior division of internal iliac artery and (ii) ovarian artery—lateral branch of abdominal artery.

Venous drainage: Into uterine venous plexus to internal iliac vein and ovarian vein.

Lymphatic drainage: Lateral aortic lymph node, internal aortic lymph node, and superficial inguinal lymph node, obturator, lateral sacral.

Nerve supply: Sympathetic from T12, and L1; parasympathetic via pelvic splanchnic nerve S2, S3, S4.

Uterus undergoes different changes in foetal condition, puberty, at pregnancy, after birth and at menopause.

Structures of uterus: Structures of uterus consist of three coats: (i) outer peritoneal coat (perimetrium), (ii) intermediate unstriped muscle (myometrium) and (iii) mucus membrane (endometrium and endocervix). The endometrium consists of surface epithelium, tubular glands and stroma; endocervix consists of columnar secretory cells and ciliated cells; glands with nonciliated secretory columnar epithelium dip into stroma.

SAQ 4 Mention the supports of uterus.

It can be classified as:

1. Supporting apparatus	Levator ani, urogenital diaphragm, perineal body.
2. Retentive apparatus	Pubocervical ligament, Mackenrodt's ligament, uterosacral ligament.
3. Holding apparatus	Broad ligament, round ligament of uterus.

LAQ 5 Describe the anatomy in brief of: (a) uterine tube and (b) ovary.

(a) Uterine tube: It is a tube on either side of uterus. Length 10 cm. For carrying ovum into uterus; laterally opens into pelvic ostium and medially into superolateral angle of the cavity of uterus. It has following parts medial to laterally: (i) pars uterine tubae, (ii) isthmus, (iii) ampulla, (iv) infundibulum from which finger-like process fimbrae projects.

Arterial supply: Uterine artery and ovarian artery.

Lymphatic drainage: Into lateral aortic, internal iliac and superficial inguinal lymph nodes. Nerve supply only sympathetic from renal and aortic plexus and pelvic plexus.

(b) Ovary: One on either side 3 cm × 2 cm × 1 cm. It contains: (i) germinal epithelium, (ii) tunica albuginea, (iii) Graafian follicles, (iv) stroma, (v) corpus luteum.

Arterial supply: Ovarian artery branch of abdominal aorta.

Venous drainage: Right ovarian vein opens into inferior vena cava and left ovarian vein opens into renal vein.

Lymphatic drainage: Into lateral aortic group of lymph node.

Develops from: Genital ridge which is condensed coelomic epithelium over mesonephros. It descends from lumbar region to pelvis by gubernaculum.

LAQ 6 Describe in brief the menstrual cycle or uterine cycle.

In female of reproductive age group, two cycles occurring simultaneously: (i) in ovary called ovarian cycle leading to maturation and rupture of ovum and another in uterus called (ii) uterine cycle or menstrual cycle.

The menstrual cycle has three phases: (a) post-menstrual proliferative phase, (b) pre-menstrual secretory phase, (c) menstrual phase.

It is customary to start counting 1st day of menstrution as 1st day of menstrual cycle.

Following menstrual phase (which lasts 4–5 days) endometrium increases in thickness, glands become wider, convoluted.

In secretory phase, glands become tortuous, hack-saw appearance. Endometrium is infiltrated with leukocytes and three layers can be distinguished in endometrium from base to surface are: (a) stratum basalis, (b) stratum spongiosum, (c) stratum compactum.

The main purpose of the all changes of uterus in uterine cycle is preparation of an imbedding site for fertilized ovum.

SAQ 7 What is placenta? Describe it.

Placenta is discoidal, deciduate, haemochorial villous type, foeto-maternal, labyrinthine organ. Diameter15–20 cm, thickness 3 cm at center weighing 500 gm. At full term, it occupies 30% of uterine wall.

LAQ 8 Mention the different female sex hormones.

Hormones	Function
Gonadotropin releasing hormone	Decapeptide, reaches pituitary to secrete gonadotropins.
Pituitary gonado-tropin	Secretes two gonadotropins: (a) follicular stimulating hormone and (b) luteinizing hormones. In pregnancy, chorionic epithelium makes LH for continuation of corpus luteum which is concerned with placental production of progesterone.
Ovarian hormones	(i) Ovarian theca cells produce oestradiol which is converted to oestrone and oestriol in liver (called oestrogen) produces changes in organ of secondary sex characters. (ii) Corpus luteum secretes progesterone, responsible for preparation of uterus for continuation of pregnancy which is oestrogen primed.

LAQ 9 How placenta is formed?

The ovum shed from ovary traverse through uterine tube gets fertilized, its zona pellucida disappears and it implants into fundus of uterus called decidua.

Trophoblast of embryo throws small finger-like projection called villi which are surrounded by maternal blood. The chronic villi are formed all over the decidua. The portion of chorion produces placenta is called chorion frondosum, rest of the chorion is called chorion laevae.

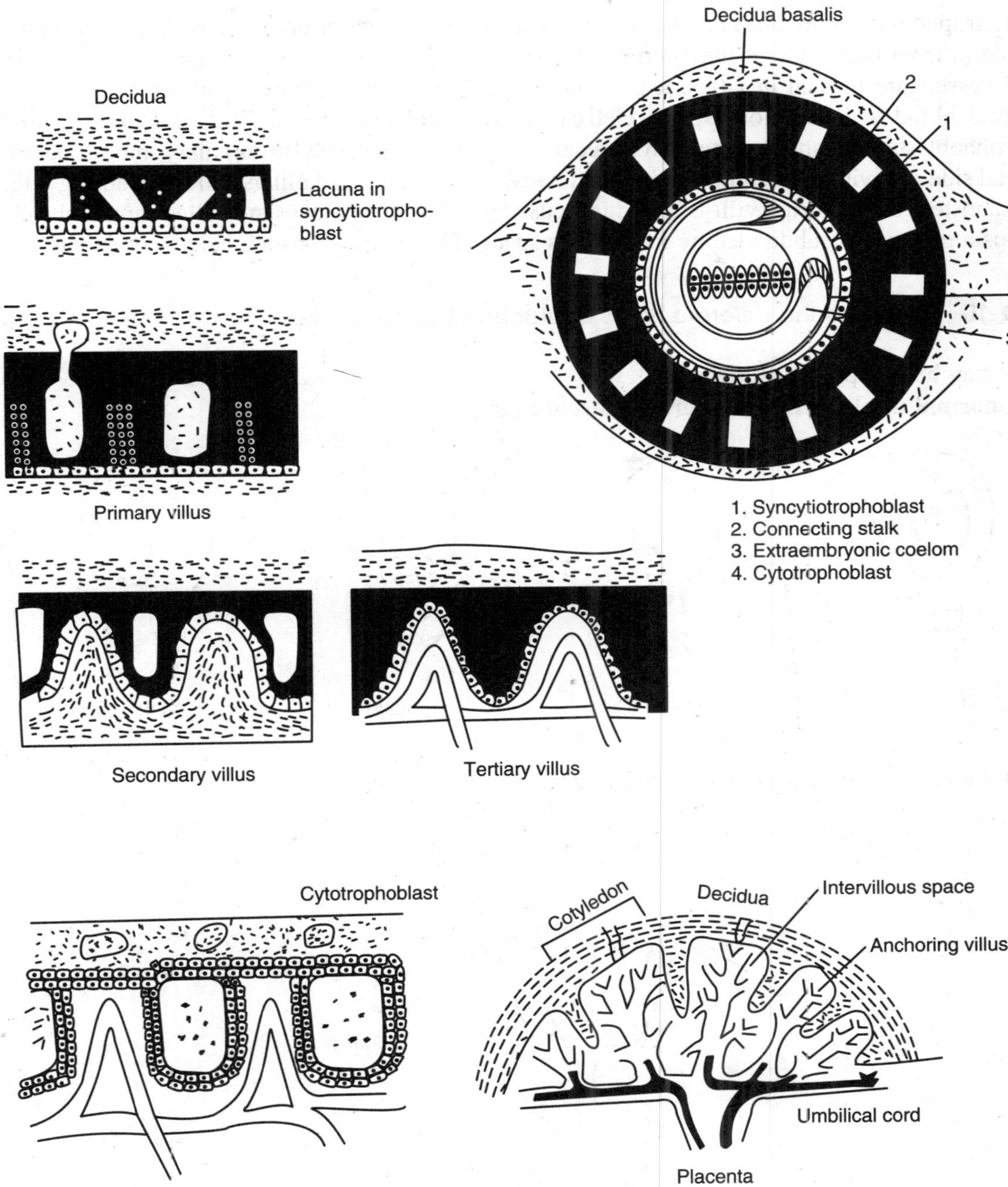

Formation of placenta

The trophoblast has two layers, outer syncytiotrophoblast and inner cytotrophoblast. Syncytiotrophoblast grows rapidly, small cavities appear within it, which arrange themselves radially called lacunae, separated by partition of syncytium called trabecullae. Endometrium is eroded and blood is filled in lacunar space.

Cytotrophoblast multiplies and grows to enter trabeculus called primary villus. Extraembryonic mesoderm from inner side of mesoderm enters primary villus to produce secondary villus, when blood vessels are formed in villus, it is tertiary villus. Foetal blood thus circulates in villus and maternal blood in intervillous space. Cells of cytotrophoblast enter the full thickness, called cytotrophoblastic shell and syncytium from deciduas. The villi are attached to the embryonic mesoderm at foetal side and with cytotrophoblastic shell on maternal side are like pillars called anchoring villi. The mainstem of anchoring villi is called truncus chroii and its branches are called ramuli chroii.

Thus a placenta is subdivided by intervillous space. The subdivisions are called cotyledons.

LAQ 10 What are the different types of placental abnormalities?

These may be grouped as following

1. Abnormal implantation in uterus (placenta previa).

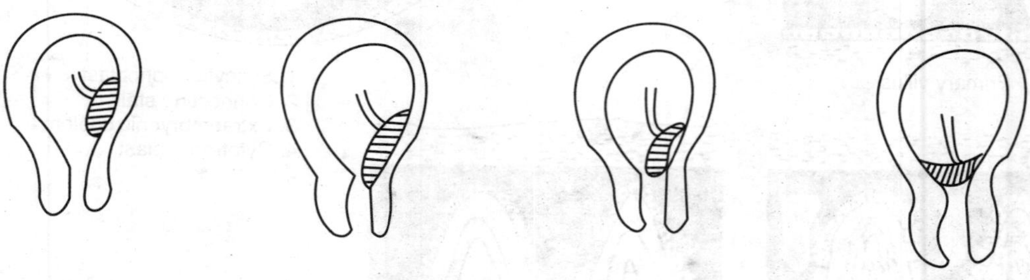

1st degree 2nd degree 3rd degree 4th degree

2. Implanted outside uterus (viz. tube, ovary, etc.).

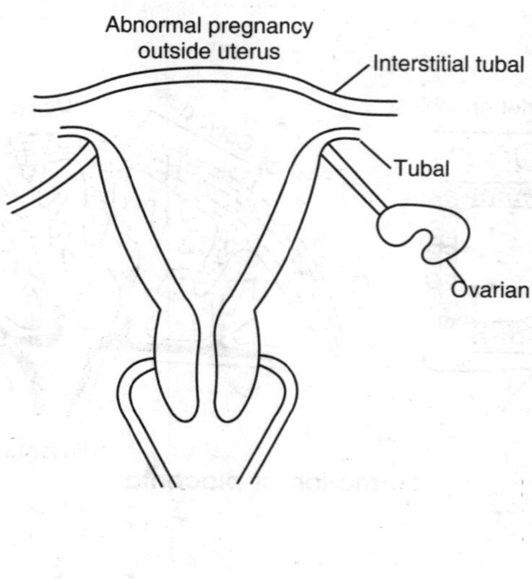

3. According to shape.

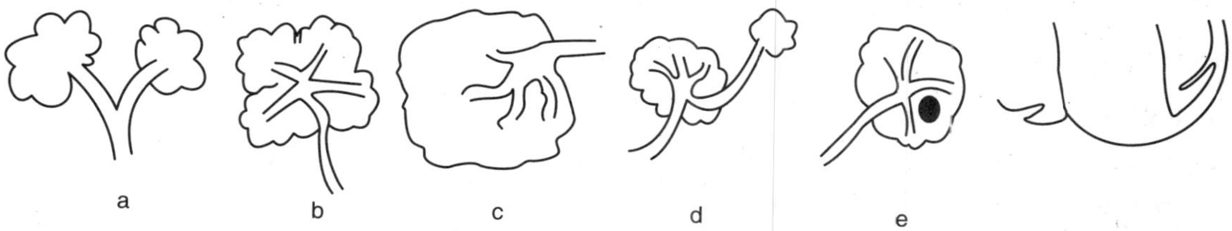

(a) Bisdiscoidal (two disc), (b) lobed, (c) diffused, (d) placenta succenturiate (small part is separated from rest), (e) fenestrated (hole in the disc), (f) circumvallated (periphery covered by fold of deciduas).

4. According to attachment of umbilical cord.

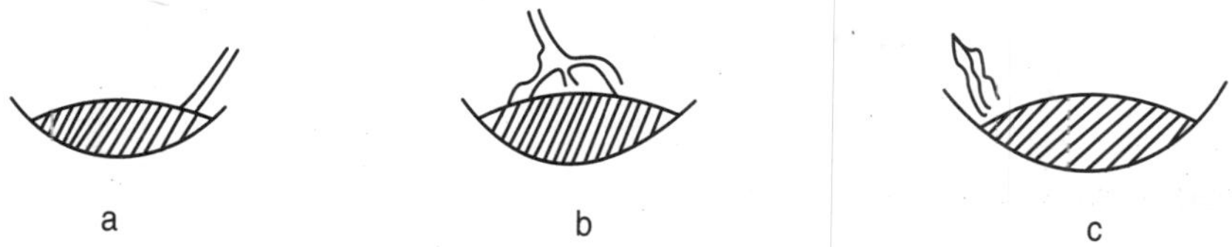

(a) Battledore (cord attached to margin), (b) furcuate (blood vessels divide before reaching placenta), (c) vilamentous insertion of placenta (blood vessels attached to amnion).

5. According to adherence.

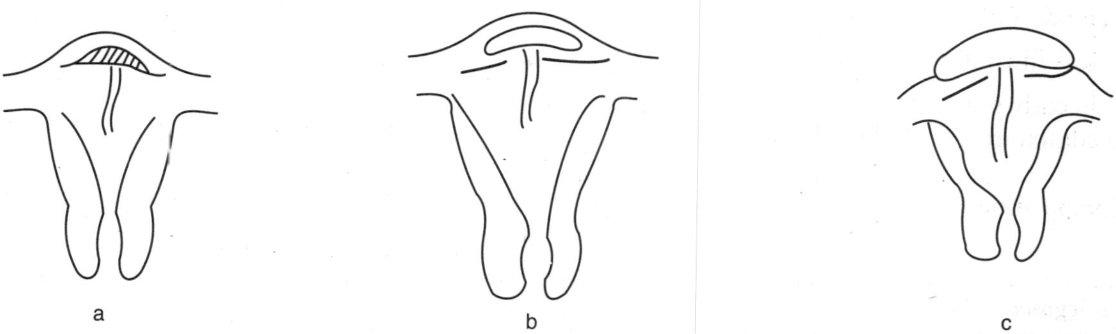

(a) Placenta accreta, (b) placenta increta, (c) placenta percreta

LAQ 11 What are the functions of placenta?

Placenta performs the following functions:

- Foetal respiratory function.
- Foetal alimentary function: Different mechanisms are: (a) diffusion (Na, K, Cl), (b) active transport (Ca, P, Fe), (c) facilitated diffusion (glucose), (d) pinocytosis (amino acids), (e) lipids and cholesterol are synthesized in foetus.
- Excretory function for foetus.
- Placenta secretes human chorionic gonadotropin, human placental lactogen, human chorionic thyrotropin, luteinising hormone releasing hormone, pregnancy specific beta glycoprotein, progesterone, oestrogen.
- Acts as foetal barrier.
- Liberates enzymes like diamine oxidase, oxytocinase, alkaline phosphatase.
- Protects foetus from immunological rejection.

SAQ 12 Name the foetal membrane.

Amnion and chorion produce inner and outer membrane of foetus.

LAQ 13 Describe the origin, physical character, composition and functions of amniotic fluid.

Regarding origin, following theories are proposed: (i) Transudate from—(a) maternal plasma, (b) foetal circulation, (ii) Secretion from amniotic epithelium, (iii) Foetus drinks about 450 ml of amniotic fluid and urinates equal amount at term daily.

It is in constant circulation and completely changed every 2.9 hours.

In early pregnancy, it is colourless gradually becomes pale yellow and after 36 weeks cloudy due to admixture of foetal epithelial cells, vernix caseosa, lunago hair.

Composition: 1. Water – 98–99% 2. Solid

Organic	Inorganic	Cells
Protein, uric acid, creatinine, glucose, lipids, hormones, PG, phospholipids, cholesterol.	pH 7.1 same as mother's plasma, but low in Na and Cl.	Cells of skin, respiratory tract, bladder, vagina, amnion, umbilical cord.

Functions

During pregnancy

- Protective for foetus, allows growth and prevents adhesion.
- Maintains temperature for foetus.
- Allows foetal movement.
- Nutritive function for foetus.
- Perhaps have immunological, biochemical, hormonal function.

During labour

- Dilates birth passage.
- Prevents placenta and foetus from damage by uterine contraction.
- Washes vagina before birth and prevents infection.

SAQ 14 What is umbilical cord?

It develops from mesoblastic tissue called body stalk connecting foetus with placenta and carrying foetal and maternal blood. It is about 50 cm long twisted spirally left to right containing: (i) amnion, (ii) Wharton jelly, (iii) two umbilical arteries and vein, (iv) remnant of allantois, vitelline duct, (v) obliterated extraembryonic coelom. No nerves. False knots may occur due to heaping up of Wharton's jelly.

2 Diagnosis of Pregnancy

LAQ 1 How the diagnosis of pregnancy is made?

The entire pregnancy is divided into three phases: (i) early (1st 12 weeks), (ii) mid (13–28 weeks), (iii) late (29–40 weeks) called 1st, 2nd and 3rd trimester, respectively.

EARLY PREGNANCY

Symptoms

- Amenorrhoea
- Morning sickness
- Constipation
- Frequency of micturition

Signs

- Breast changes:Pigmentary changes and secretion.
- Per vagina: Bluish, moist vagina and cervix soft, uterus enlarges soft elastic Hegar sign(+ve). i.e. soft and emptiness of isthmus, Palmar's sign (+ve).
- Urinary pregnancy test +ve.
- Ultrasonogram.

MID PREGNANCY

Symptoms

- Amenorrhoea.
- Enlargement of abdomen.
- Quickening from 16–20 weeks.

Signs

- Pigmentation of face, breast
- Colostrum secretion.
- Linea nigra
- Uterus felt per abdomen.
- Braxton Hicks sign.
- External and internal ballottement.
- Foetus heart sound audible.
- X-ray and ultrasound show foetus.

LATE PREGNANCY

Symptoms

- Amenorrhoea.
- Enlargement of abdomen.
- Frequency of micturition.
- Pressure symptoms.

Signs

- Cloasma.
- Oedema.
- Striae gravidarum and linea albicantes.
- FHS.

SAQ 2 What are the differential diagnoses of pregnancy?

- Full bladder
- Uterine fibroid
- Pseudocyesis
- Menopause
- Ovarian cyst

LAQ 3 Describe the different maternal physiologic changes in pregnancy.

In pregnancy, all systems undergo some changes.

1. Reproductive system:

- Uterus muscle undergoes hypertrophy and it increases in size, weight, capacity. Decidual bleeding may occur in 1st month due to implantation.
- Cervix: Hypertrophy and hyperplasia, increased vascularity, physiological leukorrhoea of pregnancy, cervical dilation due to slight increase in water, decrease in collagen fibres and glycoproteins, increase in glycosaminoglycans.
- Vagina: Excessive curd like secretion.
- Fallopian tube shows secretion, vascularity increased, hypertrophied.
- Ovary: Corpus luteum continues to grow till 2nd month, starts waning its function from 3rd month, colloid degeneration starts from 4th month, may be calcified. There is no ovulation in pregnancy, corpus luteum secretes progesterone, later placenta starts its function. This change over period is called critical phase.
- Breast: Enlarges, pigmented, secretes sticky fluid (colostrum).
- Montgomery's Tubercle enlarges. The changes are under influence of oestrogen, progesterone, human placental lactogen, anterior pituitary.

2. Cardiohaemopoietic and vascular system: Blood flow to uterus; kidneys, lungs, skin, and limb increases. Blood volume, plasma volume, red cell volume increase, but less increase in RBC and Hb of blood leading to pseudoanaemia. There is leukocytosis, rise in ESR. There is rise in fibrinogen, platelet count, factors VII, VIII, IX, X and total plasma proteins but its concentration decreases due to rise of plasma volume.

Heart: Increases in size; ECG may show left axis deviation, pulse rate and cardiac output increases.

Blood pressure in anticubital vein remain normal but femoral vein increases in normal pregnancy.

Respiratory system: Becomes diaphragmatic then thoracic. Increased inspirations, expiration, pulmonary ventilation, mucosa of respiratory tract (upper), hypernaemia, congested due to hormonal effect.

Skin changes: Pigmentation like linea nigra (xiphoid to symphysis pubis); striae gravidarum, pigmentation of areola. These pigmentations are due to hormonal effect (MSH, oestrogen) or stretching of skin.

Gastrointestinal system: Gum become vascular, nausea and vomiting may occur in early pregnancy, loss of appetite in early pregnancy, heart burn, bile stasis in liver and gallbladder.

Metabolism: Increases, body temperature rises.

- **Carbohydrate:** Increased need to meet foetal and maternal energy requirement. Fasting blood sugar is reduced for foetal utilization of glucose. Circulating insulin decreases, insulin is also destroyed by placenta. Renal threshold for glucose is lowered.
- **Lipid:** 3–4 kg stored as depot in abdominal wall, thigh, breast, serum cholesterol rises. Glycogen store decreases, prone to ketosis.
- **Protein:** Blood urea nitrogen decreases, improved protein absorption, positive nitrogen balance, serum uric acid and creatinine remain normal in spite of rise due to haemodilution.
- **Iron:** Deficiency is common,
- **Water:** There is about 6.5 kg of water retention leading to weight gain.
- **Electrolyte**: 20 gm Na; 10 gm K and chloride are retained distributed in mother and foetus due to aldosterone, ADH; estrogen and progesterone.

Renin, angiotensin, aldosterone level rises.

Gain in weight: In full course, there is 10–12 kg of weight gain in pregnancy.

Reproductive weight gain in pregnancy

Foetus, placenta, amniotic fluid, breast.

Maternal weight gain

Maternal store of protein, fat, water.

- **Endocrine system:** HCG can be detected in maternal urine, some crosses over foetal blood. It comprises α and β subunits of peptide chain. Human placental lactogen (HPL) rises up to 36 weeks, human chorionic thyrotropin (HCT) secreted by placental trophoblast. LHRH secreted by cytotrophoblast. Progesterone secreted by corpus luteum up to 6th week and placenta from 5th week. Estrogen: 20 different estrogens are demonstrated in pregnant woman. Aldosterone and plasma cortisol level rises. Protein hormone relaxin is released to relax pelvic joints and cervical dilatation.

Pituitary, thyroid, parathyroid glands show enlargement, but there is little morphological change in adrenal cortex.

Nervous system: Neuritis, vitamin B deficiency, carpal tunnel syndrome, irritability, depression, emotional outburst, pervertion of appetite (longings) sciatica syndrome.

Locomotor system: Backache, lumbar lordosis with waddling gait.

3 Antenatal Care

SAQ 1 What do you mean by gravida and para?

Gravida is state of pregnancy, irrespective of age of viability of foetus. Para is state of woman who bore after baby is viable.

SAQ 2 What do you mean by high-risk pregnancies?

These are cases with complications of mortality and morbidity for mother and her unborn child requires intensive antenatal care. The factors are:

Obstetric factors

- All primigravida and grand-multipara.
- Age above 35 and below 19
- Height less than 145 cm.
- Bad obstetric history.
- Disproportionate pelvis.
- Malpresentation.
- Threatened abortion, Hypertension, toxemia.
- Rh incompatibility.
- Premature labour.
- Post-maturity.

Medical factors

- Anaemia.
- Malnutrition
- Hypertension.
- Tuberculosis
- Obesity.
- Thyroid diseases.
- Hepatitis
- Syphilis.

Social factors

- Unemployed.
- Illeteracy.
- Poor habits.
- Social customs and beliefs.

SAQ 3 What is Naegel's rule?

Expected date of delivery (EDD) is estimated. The first day of last menstrual period plus nine calender months and seven days is expected day of delivery as per the rule.

LAQ 4 Describe in brief the format of antenatal check up.

A. (i) History, (ii) identification (name, age, gravida, parity), (iii) social history married/single/widow; education, occupation and income of wife and husband; religion; Hindu/Muslim/others, (iv) medical history, (v) chief complaints in chronological order, (vi) menstrual history menarche, duration in days, amount of blood loss; LMP; EDD, (vii) obstetric history: each past pregnancies, (viii) contraceptive history, (ix) dietetic history veg/nonveg, (x) past history and drug intake, (xi) family history of hypertension, diabetes, tuberculosis.

B. Physical examination: Height, weight, nutrition, built, anemia, jaundice, clubbing, oedema, thyroid, pulse, BP, palpation of liver, spleen, kidney, teeth, heart, chest.

C. Obstetric examination: (i) Breast, (ii) per abdomen height of uterus, (iii) per vagina (examination should be done in presence of reliable third person nurse, with proper consent with aseptic precaution, vulva, vagina, pelvic organs are examined, (iv) per rectal examination.

D. Laboratory tests: TC/DC/ESR/Hb%/ABO; Rh group, VDRL; urine analysis, pregnancy test, cervical cytology by PAP stain; cervical smear; routine stool examination.

SAQ 5 What are the purposes of antenatal check up?

- To diagnose pregnancy
- Health screening
- Genetic counseling
- Contraceptive advice.

SAQ 6 What are the important causes of rise in fundal height in relation to amenorrhoea?

These are:

- Wrong date of LMP
- Hydromnios
- Twin pregnancy
- IUFD
- Pelvic tumor
- Malpresentation
- Growth retardation.

SAQ 7 What are the different methods of estimating gestational age?

The different methods to estimate the gestational age are as follows:

(i) Fundal height, (ii) McDonald's rule: $\frac{\text{Height of fundus in cm} \times 8}{7} = $ Duration of pregnancy in week.

SAQ 8 How the height of uterus corresponds with different periods of pregnancy clinically?

The height of uterus corresponds in the following way:

(i) At 12 weeks, uterus becomes abdominal organ from pelvis.

(ii) At 24 weeks, uterus lies at umbilicus.

(iii) At 16 weeks, lower one-third of umbilicus and symphysis pubis.

(iv) At 20 weeks, upper two-thirds of umbilicus and symphysis pubis.

(v) At 36 weeks, at of xiphisternum.

(vi) At 28 weeks, lower one-third of xiphisternal and umbilicus.

(vii) At 32 weeks, upper one-third of xiphisterum and umbilicus.

(viii) At 40 weeks, comes down from xiphisterum but lies above 32 weeks due to engagement of head.

SAQ 9 What are the principles of antenatal advice?

Principles of antenatal advice are:

- To motivate for antenatal check up at regular interval
- Advice for diet and personal hygine
- To immunize against tetanus
- To prepare mind for childbirth and motivate family planning.

SAQ 10 When to give tetanus toxoid to pregnant women?

At 20, 24, and 28 weeks of pregnancy.

SAQ 11 What are the indications of ultrasound in pregnancy?

These are:

- Diagnosis of early pregnancy.
- Abortion.
- Incomplete abortion.
- Multiple pregnancy.
- Ectopic pregnancy.
- Hydatidiform mole.

First half of pregnancy

• Doppler apparatus for FHS in 2nd half of pregnancy. • Foetal cephalometry (biparietal diameter). • Small for dates. • Location of placenta. • Multiple pregnancy with presentation. • Foetal abnormalities. • IUFD. • Fibroid, ovarian tumor.	2nd half of pregnancy

SAQ 12 What is the relative safety of ultrasound in pregnancy?

It is a safe procedure, if better standardization is made and peak intensity kept low.

SAQ 13 What conditions can be diagnosed by X-rays in pregnancy?

X-ray is better to be avoided in pregnancy because of radiation hazard and better, safe diagnostic procedure, are available. The condition which can be diagnosed by X-ray in pregnancy are:

- Foetus skeleton is visualized at 16th weeks.
- Spalding sign (overlapping of foetus cranial vault) suggest IUFD.
- Lateral X-ray during labour is valuable for trailing of labour.
- X-ray placentography.

SAQ 14 When to suggest X-ray of chest in pregnancy?

X-ray of chest suggests in pregnancy:

- Personal history of tuberculosis
- Recent family history of contact of TB.
- Immigrants
- Diabetics
- Living in bad home conditions
- PUO; unexplained respiratory symptoms
- Recent tuberculin conversion.

LAQ 15 Name some special tests to monitor foetus in pregnancy.

(I) Testing foetoplacental unit by amniocentesis

- **Hormones**
  - Oestrogen.
  - HPL.
- **Enzymes**
  - Heat stable Alkaline phosphates
- **Other**
  - α - fetoprotein.
  - Chromosomes.
  - Blood pigments.
  - Urea; creatinine.
  - LSAR for maturity. (lecithin sphingomyelin area ratio)

(II) Physical properties foetus and mother

- Uterine size of mother.
- Weight gain of mother
- Foetal movement.
- Ultrasound cephalometry.

(III) Stress test

- Oxytocin test uteroplacental unit.
- Hypoxia, monitor foetal heart

SAQ 16 What are the indications of amniocentesis?

These may be grouped into:

AMINIOCENTESIS

Therapeutic

- In hydramnios to stabilize induction.
- Intrauterine transfusion.
- Induction of labour by urea or PG in 2nd trimester.

Diagnostic

- To determine foetal maturity.
- Chromosomal analysis.
- Enzyme analysis to determine chromosome disorder.
- Alfa-fetoprotein to determine neural tube defect.

Haemorrhage in Early Pregnancy

4

SAQ 1 What are the causes of haemorrhage in early pregnancy?

Causes of bleeding up to 28 weeks are:
- Abortion
- Hydatidiform mole
- Disturbance of ectopic pregnancy
- Cervical polyp
- Cervical cancer
- Bleeding disorders of mother
- Abortion contributes the major cause.

SAQ 2 What is abortion?

It is the expulsion of product of conception before the foetus become viable, i.e. 28 weeks of pregnancy. It is miniature labour with signs of onset(threatened abortion) followed by dilatation of cervix and expulsion of conceptus. A miniature puerperium follows it.

LAQ 3 What are the causes of abortion?

It may be classified as:

Spontaneous abortion

(i) Fault in the embryo development (chromosomal defect).

(ii) Fault in maternal environment.
- Maternal disease
- Infection
- Trauma
- Hormonal deficiency
- Cervical incompetence
- Retroversion.

Induced abortion

(i) MTP
(ii) Criminal abortion.

SAQ 4 What is habitual abortion?

This is spontaneous, recurrent abortion on three or more times.

SAQ 5 What are the varieties of spontaneous abortion?

These are:

Spontaneous abortion

Threatened abortion	Inevitable abortion	Incomplete abortion	Complete abortion	Septic abortion	Missed abortion
Pregnancy continuation is possible.	Process of expulsion of conceptus is inevitable	Expulsion process is incomplete.	Expulsion process is complete.	There is sepsis of conceptus and uterus.	Ovum is dead and retained in uterus.

SAQ 6 What are the grades of septic abortion?

- Grade I infection up to myometrium
- Grade II infection up to pelvic structure
- Grade III infection spreading to peritoneum

SAQ 7 What is blood mole/fleshy mole/tuberous mole/carneous mole?

In case of missed abortion within 12 weeks, the product of conception may turn into ovoid, tough, fleshy mass due to slow, progressive haemorrhage in choriodecidual space and amniotic sac is surrounded by firm laminated blood clot, embryo may shrink or absent and may remain inside uterus for long.

SAQ 8 What are the dangers of abortions?

Dangers of abortion may be grouped into:

Immediate

- Haemorrhage
- Shock
- Injury to uterus and viscera
- Anuria
- Coagulation defects
- Sepsis

Late

- Placental polyp
- PID
- Ill health
- Choriocarcinoma

LAQ 9 How will you manage threatened, incomplete and inevitable abortion?

They are managed as described below:

Threatened abortion	Inevitable abortion	Incomplete abortion
Principle: ***Try to conserve pregnancy***	***Evacuate the uterus***	***Evacuate the uterus***
Advice: (i) Rest, (ii) Sedation with phenobarbitone or diazepam. (iii) Uterine relaxatant, isoxsuprine, ritrodine, etc. (iv) Hormone 17 alpha hydroxy progesterone caproate (proluton depot) (IM), or tab allesternol 5 mg. (gestanin) orally TDS. If HCG level is 20,000 IU in 55–110 days outcome is good but if less than 10,000 IU then outcome is poor.	General treatment IV fluid (5% dextrose). Blood transfusion, Inj. morphine, Inj. ergometrine. Local treatment up to 12 weeks: Dilatation and curettage after 12 wks Syntocinon drip 10–20 units with 500 ml of 5% dextrose or abdominal hysterotomy.	Dilatation and curettage.

SAQ 10 Name the organism generally involved in septic abortion and its treatment.

Gram-positive: Sterpto, Staphylo, Cl. welchii

Gram-negative: Proteus; E.coli; Bacteroids.

Investigations: TC/DC/ESR/urinalysis, blood sugar; bilirubin, urine for culture; blood fibrinogen, blood group; X-ray chest and pelvis, electrolytes, urine output.

Treatment: (i) Antibiotics, (ii) plenty of drinks and nourishing diet, (iii) if infection restricted to uterus than surgical evacuation of uterus, (iv) uterus severely injured and infected then laparotomy hysterectomy; pelvic abscess draining by colpotomy. Septic shock is treated with: (i) IV fluid, (ii) hydrocortisone, (iii) AGS, (iv) antibiotics.

SAQ 11 How will you treat missed abortion?

(i) Wait and watch up to 6 weeks with clot observation fibrinogen estimation and platelet count.
(ii) IV syntocinon or PGE2 vaginal suppository.
(iii) Dilatation and curettage up to 12 weeks.
(iv) Above 12 weeks if induction fails then hysterectomy is done.

SAQ 12 What are the indications and contraindications of Shirodkar and McDonald's operation?

These are operation performed on habitual aborter with: (i) cervical incompetence in 2nd trimester or (ii) early third trimester in premature labour.

Contraindication: (i) Haemorrhage (early or mid pregnancy) (ii) uterine tetany, (iii) hydromnios or rupture of hydromnios.

In Shirodkar operation under general anaesthesia, a nonabsorbable encircling suture is placed around internal os underneath covering mucosa.

In McDonald's operation under general anaesthesia, a purse string nonabsorbable suture is placed at the junction of vagina and cervix.

SAQ 13 What is legal abortion?

The legal abortion or MTP or therapeutic abortion is deliberate, induced abortion to safe the woman from the risks and mortality of criminal abortion.

LAQ 14 What are the scopes and indications of MTP?

MTP act (1971) starts operating whole of India except JK gives direction for person who can perform it, place where it can be performed and indications of performing it.

Indication

- Maternal diseases
- Social cause
  - Contraceptive failure
  - Pregnancy by rape
  - Unplanned pregnancy
- Eugenic cause
  - Malformation of foetus

SAQ 15 What are the different methods of performing MTP?

Different methods adopted for performing MTP are as follows:

Up to 6–12 weeks

- Suction evacuation
- D and C

13–20 weeks of pregnancy

- 20% saline aminotransfusion
- 40% urea aminotransfusion
- Extra-amniotic ethacridine
- Hysterotomy

SAQ 16 Describe the clinical feature of Hydatidiform mole.

Generally above 45 years of age, presents with pain abdomen and recurrent vaginal bleeding and expulsion of grape-like vesicles, vomiting, eclampsia.

Signs of anaemia, early pregnancy, large uterus (soft, cystic, without foetal movement, os closed bilateral cystic ovaries).

Investigation:

(i) HCG raised, oestrogen and placental lactogen low.

(ii) Radiography (foetus; chest X-ray; HSG)

(iii) Ultrasonography.

SAQ 17 What complications may arise out of MTP?

Following complications may arise out of MTP:

Immediate complications	Late complications
• Uterine perforation	• Recurrent abortion
• Haemorrhage	• Perinatal death
• Injury of cervix	• Premature birth
• Infection	• PID
• Embolism	• Ectopic pregnancy
• Hypernatraemia	• Infertility
• Anaesthetic hazards	• Endometriosis
• Coagulation defect	

SAQ 18 What is hydatidiform mole?

Hydatidiform mole/vasicular mole/gestational trophoblastic disease is one of the important cause of haemorrhage in early pregnancy where chorionic villi are transformed, into translucent mass like hydatid cyst, clinically it may be: (i) hydatidiform mole, (ii) invasive mole, (iii) choriocarcinoma.

Appearance

Macroscopic

Numerous vesicle of different sizes delicate, pediculate, lutein cyst may be seen in ovary due to excess HCG

Microscopic

There is proliferation of cyto- and syncytoblast, hydropic degeneration and degenerated nuclei. Villi filled with fluid. Blood vessels of villi are obliterated. Decidua may show inflammatory reaction (syncytical endometritis). When it burrows the uterus (invasive mole), choriocarcinoma or chorioepithelioma is malignant tumour of chorionic trophoblast.

SAQ 19 What are the differential diagnosis of hydatidiform mole?

They are as below:

- Threatened abortion
- Hydramnios
- Multiple pregnancy
- Ovarian cyst
- Fibroid
- Retroverted gravid uterus
- Distended bladder

SAQ 20 Mention some important complications of hydatidiform mole.

They are:

- Haemorrhage
- Perforation of uterus
- Infection
- Malignancy (choriocarcinoma).

SAQ 21 What is the principle of treatment of hydatidiform mole?

Early evacuation after diagnosis and follow up for detection of malignancy by urinary HCG test by immunoassay. If HCG values are high (rule out pregnancy) after 6 weeks, suggests choriocarcinoma or invasive mole. They present with subinvoluted uterus with recurrent vaginal haemorrhage. Histology from uterine curettage, should be done, chest X-ray may show cannon ball if there is metastasis.

5 Ectopic Pregnancy

SAQ 1 What is ectopic pregnancy?

Pregnancy outside the normal uterine cavity is ectopic pregnancy, viz.

- Tubal ampulla; isthmus/interstitial
- Ovary
- Cornual
- Abdominal

SAQ 2 What is tubal mole?

It is chorio-tubal haemorrhage separating and killing the ovum. The gestational sac from surrounding wall. The dead ovum surrounded by layers of blood clot.

SAQ 3 How the tubal pregnancy is terminated?

Tubal pregnancy is terminated in one of the following ways:

- Tubal mole
- Tubal abortion
- Tubal rupture producing (paratubal or pelvic haematocele, haematoma broad ligament)
- Secondary abdominal pregnancy (leading to spurious labour, infection, mummification of foetus or lithopaedion due to salt deposition, may die and absorbed).

SAQ 4 Mention some differential diagnoses of tubal pregnancy.

Acute: Salpingitis; abortion; ovarian cyst; appendicitis.

Chronic: Retroverted gravid uterus; fibroid; TO mass, loaded rectum; ovarian cyst.

LAQ 5 Describe the clinical features of tubal pregnancy.

Clinical features of tubal pregnancy is mentioned as below:

Acute type

Symptoms

- Amenorrhoea
- Pain of lower abdomen
- Vaginal discharge
- Fainting attack

Signs

- Anemia and shock
- Tender abdomen
- Cullen's sign
- Vaginal tenderness
- Frank blood in pouch of Douglas
- USG and laparotomy confirms.

Chronic type

Symptoms

- Amenorrhoea
- Pain abdomen
- Vaginal discharge
- Faints
- Expulsion of decidual cyst

Signs

- Fever
- Tender abdomen
- Uterus bulky
- Tenderness on
- P/V and P/R
- Pregnancy test positive
- Leukocytosis USG and laparoscopy confirms diagnosis.

SAQ 6 How will you manage tubal pregnancy?

They are managed in the following ways:

(i) Hospitalization
(ii) Inj. morphine and atropine
(iii) IV fluid
(iv) Quick laparotomy with salpingectomy
(v) Blood transfusion or autohaemotransfusion
(vi) If patient wants sterilization then tubectomy

For chronic type laparotomy, salpingectomy with gestational sac.

Rh negative mother given 100 μg RhD gamma globulin. For abdominal pregnancy – laparotomy and removal of gestational sac.

Antepartum Haemorrhage

6

SAQ 1 Define antepartum haemorrhage (APH).

It is bleeding from genital tract after 28 weeks, but before delivery.

SAQ 2 What are the causes of APH?

- Placenta praevia
- Accidental haemorrhage
- APH with indeterminate origin
- Cervical polyp
- Cervical cancer
- Varicose vein of vagina

SAQ 3 What is placenta praevia?

Here placenta is implanted in lower uterine segment partially or completely. Occurs in 1 in 200 deliveries, may be grouped in four degrees 1st degree (lateral placenta previa) occupying upper part of lower uterine segment. 2nd degree (marginal placenta previa) placenta reaches up to margin of internal OS. 3rd degree (incomplete placenta previa) placenta covers internal OS when it is closed. 4th degree (central placenta previa) covers the internal as even when it is closed. It may be anterior or posterior in 1st and 2nd degrees. The posterior placenta previa interferes with engagements and produces more haemorrhage.

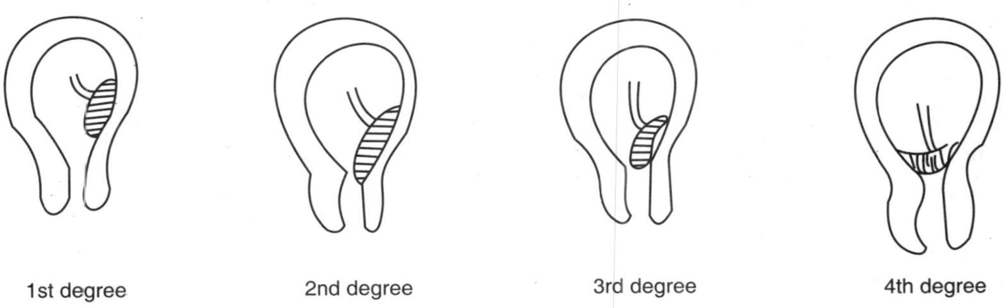

SAQ 4 Whose blood is lost from placenta praevia?

The mother's blood is lost mostly.

SAQ 5 What are causes of bleeding placenta praevia?

(i) Detachment of non-elastic placenta by dilating uterine segment, (ii) coitus.

SAQ 6 How the placenta previa presents?

Placenta praevia presents in the following ways:

Symptoms

Recurrent painless causeless bleeding P/V.

Signs

Signs of pregnancy, shock, anaemia, malpresentation (high floating)

> No per vagina examination should be performed. It can only be performed in OT if caesarean section can be performed there.

SAQ 7 What are the different ways to localize placenta?

Direct

- Soft tissue radiograph
- Displacement radiograph
- Ultrasonography.

Indirect

- Cystography
- Amniography
- Thermography
- Aortography.

SAQ 8 What are the risks of placenta praevia?

The risks of placenta previa are as following:

Maternal

- Haemorrhage(ante-, intra- and postpartum)
- Shock
- Sepsis
- Embolism
- Rupture uterus.

Foetal

- Prematurity
- Asphyxia
- Malformation
- Birth trauma

LAQ 9 How you will manage placenta previa?

It should be treated in hospital where infrastructure for caesarean section is available.

Patient not in labour

- Improve anemia and try to advance pregnancy, if bleeding has ceased.
- At 38 weeks, expected treatment ends.

Patient in labour

1. Vaginal bleeding is active:
(a) Low rupture of membrane if placenta previa 1° and 2° anterior or by, (b) Willett's scalp traction forceps. In 3rd stage of labour, Inj. ergometrine 0.5 mg IV after birth of foetal head and oxytocin 5 IU by IV drip. Placenta acreta if present is another danger.

SAQ 10 What is abruptio placenta/ablatio placenta/accidental haemorrhage?

In abruptio placenta, the normally situated placenta in upper segment are prematurely separated. There are three clinical varieties:

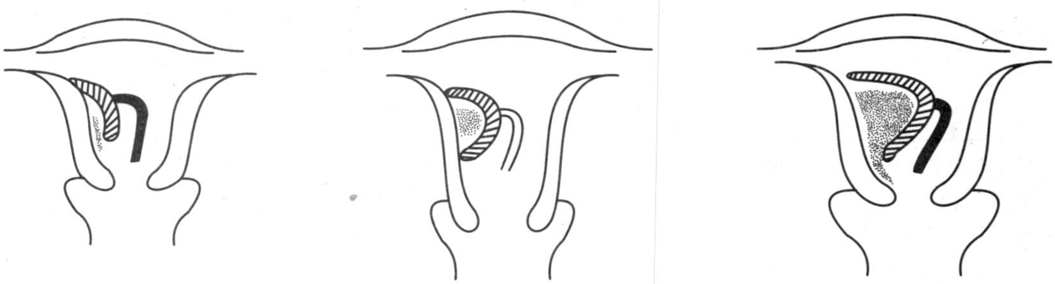

(i) Revealed (ii) Concealed (iii) Mixed type

SAQ 11 What is Page's classification of abruptio placenta?

Abruptio placentae are classified into following four grades:

Grade - 0	Grade - I	Grade - II	Grade - III
• Detected after delivery	• No shock • Mild uterine tetany and bleeding	• Foetal distress. • Bleeding and tetany • No shock	• Shock • IUFD • Coagulation failure • Uterine tetany

SAQ 12 What are the causes of abruptio placenta?

- Toxaemia
- Trauma
- Grandemultipara
- Anemia
- Folic acid deficiency
- Compression of inferior vena cava by gravid uterus

SAQ 13 What are the differences between abruptio placenta and placenta previa?

In abruptio placenta, bleeding is concealed or revealed, painful; toxemia is often present. Uterus is firm and hard; foetus felt with difficulties placenta in upper segment.

In placenta previa, reveal painless vaginal bleeding, toxemia generally not present, uterus is elastic soft with abnormal foetal presentation, placenta in lower uterine segments.

LAQ 14 How will you manage accidental haemorrhage?

Patient should be hospitalized.

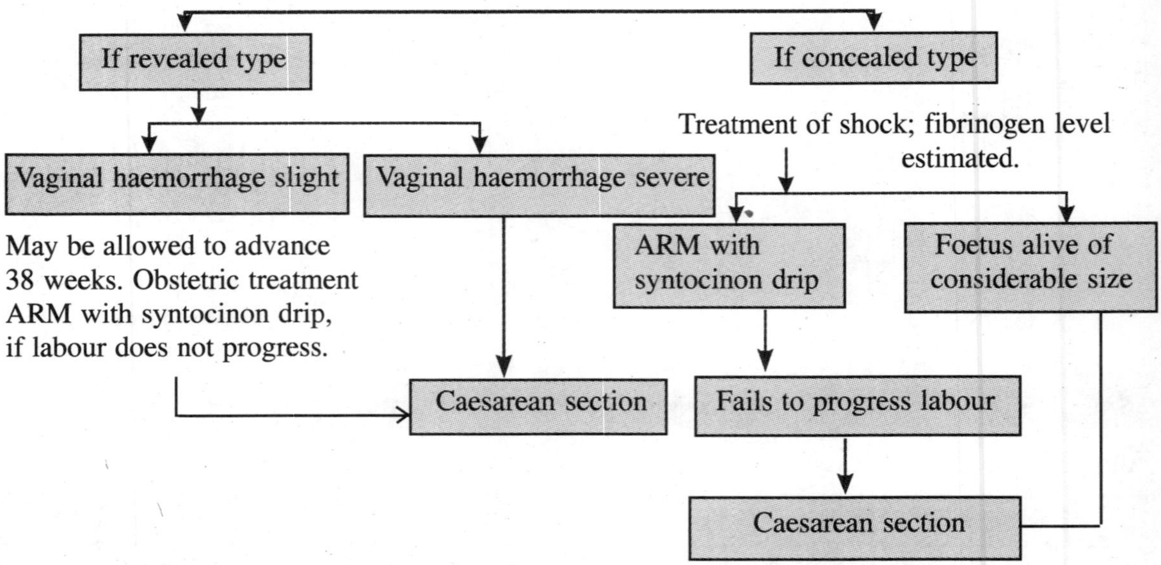

Third stage of labour should be treated properly with close observation of puerperium.

7 Toxaemias of Pregnancy

SAQ 1 What are the different etiologies of hypertensive disorder of pregnancy?

These are:

- Pregnancy-induced hypertension
- Gestational hypertension
- Essential hypertension
- Chronic renal disease

SAQ 2 What is pre-eclampsia?

This syndrome generally occurs after 20 weeks of pregnancy presented with: (i) Persistent high blood pressure above 140/90 mm Hg. (ii) Proteinuria or oedema or both. The first signs to appear are oedema then hypertension then proteinuria.
The diagnosis and treatment should be started early.

LAQ 3 What are the important theories of pre-eclampsia?

- Placental toxin theory: Infarcted placenta releases hysterotin, thromboplastin, etc. producing pre-eclampsia.
- Disturbances of nutrition (over or under).
- Excess antidiuretic hormone and water poisoning.
- Hypoproteinaemic theory.
- Immune response.
- Endocrine dysfunction.
- Hyperplacentosis (hydatidiform mole, hydrops foetalis, diabetes mellitus).
- Uterorenal reflex due to overdistension of uterus produces renal cortical ischaemia responsible for signs of pre-eclampsia.

LAQ 4 What are the clinical features of pre-eclampsia?

The clinical features of pre-eclampsia are as mentioned below:

Symptoms

- May be diagnosed on routine check-up or oedema of feet
- Headach
- Insomnia
- Dizziness of vision
- Oliguria
- Epigastric pain

Signs

- Pregnancy above 20 weeks
- Weight gain
- Hypertension
- Oedema
- Proteinuria
- Ophthalmoscopic exam
  — Retinal arterioles constriction
  — Oedema of optic disc
  — Haemorrhage
  — Cotton wool exudate
  — Detachment
  — Nicking of veins where it is crossed by arterioles.

SAQ 5 What is role over test?

A pregnant woman beyond 28–32 weeks of pregnancy rests on left lateral position for 15 minutes for stable BP recording. She is turned to supine position and BP is recorded within 2–5 minutes. If the diastolic BP is more than 20 mm Hg then Gant claimed it is diagnostic to predict pre-eclampsia.

SAQ 6 What are the different tests for proteinuria?

- Heat test with acetic acid
- Salicylsulfonic acid test (5 ml of urine + 25 drops of 25% sulicylsulfuric acid produces turbidity)
- Reagent strips
- Esbach's quantitative test.

SAQ 7 Mention the important investigation of pre-eclampsia.

- Urine examination
- Ophthalmoscopic examination
- Blood for TC/DC/ESR/Hb%/uric acid/urea/creatinine
- Test to evaluate foetal status of uterus.

LAQ 8 What are the complications of pre-eclampsia?

Complications of pre-eclampsia are:

Recent or immediate

- Eclampsia
- IUFD
- Accidental haemorrhage
- Eye and cerebral complications
- Coagulation failure
- Growth retardation with premature birth
- PPH
- Postpartum shock.

Remote

- Hypertension
- Chronic nephritis
- Recurrent pre-eclampsia

SAQ 9 Mention the important differential diagnoses of pre-eclampsia.

The pre-eclampsia has to be differentiated from:

- Nephritis
- Essential hypertension
- Severe anaemia
- Coarctation of aorta
- Pheochromocytoma

LAQ 10 How to manage pre-eclampsia?

This may be managed in the following ways:

- Rest
- Low Na and protein diet
- Fluid up to 1.5 liters
- Drugs like frusemide; diazepam or phenobarbitone, severe hypertension is treated with adelphane aldomet, β-blockers
- Obstetric treatment – (a) may be spontaneous labour, (b) induction of labour by syntocinon 5 IU with 5% of 540 ml of dextrose IV (c) elective caesarean section indications (closed os; elderly primi; overdated pregnancy; CPD; IUGR).

SAQ 11 What is eclampsia?

The syndrome of eclampsia presents with:

- Hypertension
- Proteinuria

- Oedema along with epileptiform convulsion. The eclampsia is preceded by pre-eclampsia. The causes of convulsion are cerebral hypoxia due to arteriolar spasm, cerebral oedema and cerebral dysarrhythmia. The convulsion may be antepartum, intrapartum or postpartum commonly in primigravidae.

SAQ 12 Name the important differential diagnoses of eclampsia.

- Epilepsy
- Hysteria
- CVA
- Strychnine poisoning
- SOL of brain
- Meningitis

LAQ 13 Describe the clinical features of eclampsia.

Clinical features of eclampsia can be grouped into four stages:

Premonitory stage	Tonic stage	Clonic stage	Stage of coma
Twitching of hands, face, rolling of eyes, head drawn to one side, unconscious – last 30 seconds.	Whole body goes into spasm, tongue protrudes, cyanosed respiration ceases, last-30 second.	Muscles of body relax and contracts, blood and froth comes out of nose and mouth, cyanosis gradually disappears, last for—minute.	Slight to deep, may be followed by another fit.

SAQ 14 What are the clinical types of eclampsia?

These are:

1. Fulminating: Sudden eclampsia without warnings.
2. Insidious: Convulsion in earlier diagnosed pre-eclampsia.
3. Eclampsia without convulsion: Coma.
4. Intercurrent – Pregnancy continuing with control of fits.

SAQ 15 What are the causes of maternal mortality in eclampsia?

- CVA
- CCF
- Asphyxia
- Renal failure

- Bronchopneumonia
- Puerperal sepsis
- Respiratory failure
- Postpartum shock

SAQ 16 What are the principles of management of eclampsia?

These are:

1. Control of fits.
2. Control of BP
3. Management of complications.
4. Termination of pregnancy.

LAQ 17 How will you treat eclampsia?

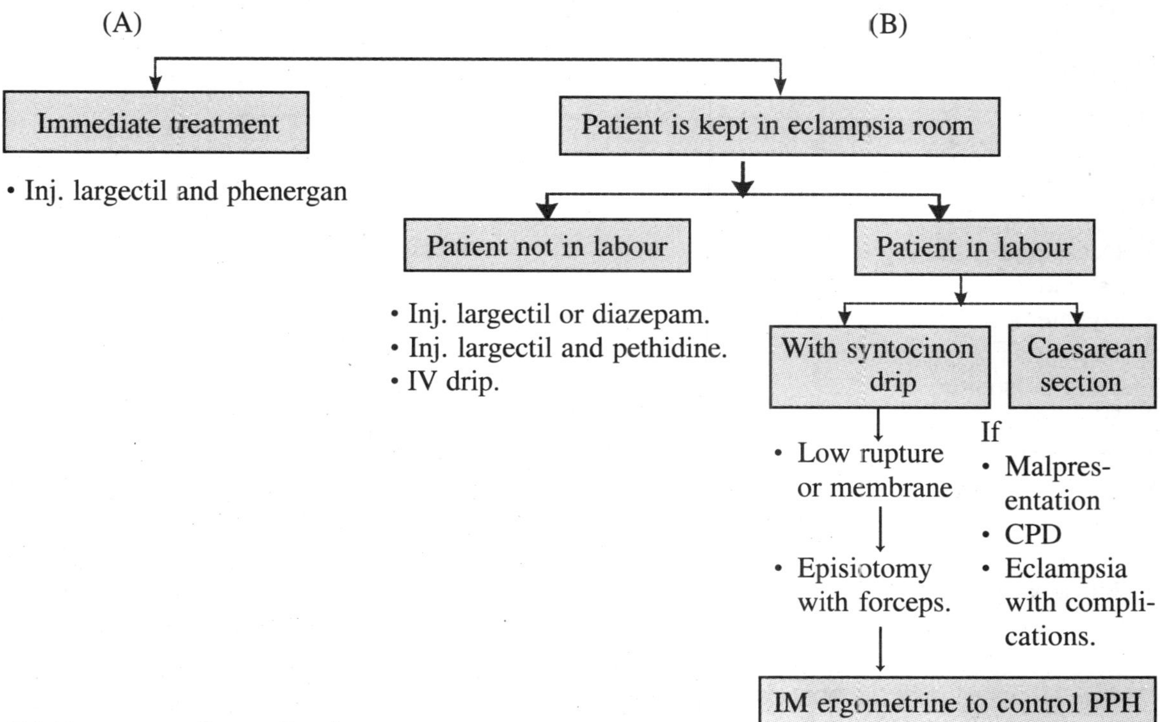

(C) Treatment of complications:

- *Heart failure:* Lasix; digoxin,
- *Pulmonary oedema:* Lasix, O_2 inhalation,
- *Oliguria:* Hypertonic glucose.

8 Some Diseases in Pregnancy

SAQ 1 What is morning sickness?

This symptom is generally found in primigravida, absent in subsequent pregnancies, usually in 2nd month, presents with nausea ending in vomiting after rising or first meal. There is no discomfort after vomiting and no suppression of appetite.

LAQ 2 What are the causes of vomiting in pregnancy?

This can be grouped as follows:

Vomiting in 1st half of pregnancy

- Occasional vomiting is common in 1st and 2nd month
- Hyperemesis gravidarum
- Hepatitis
- Food poisoning
- Worms
- Pyelonephritis
- Ovarian cyst twisted
- Gastritis
- Volvulus
- Intestinal obstruction.

Vomiting in 2nd half of pregnancy

- Occasional slight vomiting is common
- Pre-eclampsia
- Hydramnios (acute)
- Ketosis
- Hydatidiform mole
- Hysteria
- Diabetes

SAQ 3 What is hyperemesis gravidarum?

It is excessive vomiting in early months of pregnancy causing deterioration of the health of the mother. All swallowed are rejected and vomited out with bile staining fluid leading to carbohydrate starvation, glycogen depletion, ketosis develops, pulse rate increases, weight reduces, sleeplessness, furred tongue, twitching of muscles, epigastric pain, scanty urine (with albumin, blood and cast) temperature rises, loss of memory, convulsion, coma, peripheral neuritis.

SAQ 4 What are the causes of hyperemesis gravidarum?

The possible theories of its genesis are:

1. Neurosis theory
2. Endocrine theory (excess of chorionic gonadotropin and oestrogen)

LAQ 5 How you with manage hyperemesis gravidarum?

This can be managed as follows:

- Isolation in hospital
- Diet mainly carbohydrate to start with gradually to normal diet
- IV fluids
- Drugs: (a) sedative diazepam; largectil, (b) antiemetics (meclizine, prochlorperazine; trifluoromazine, promethazine), (c) vitamin B and vitamin C: B_6
- Care of bowel, oral hygine, emesis chart
- Obstetric care, if patient fails to improve, termination of pregnancy.

SAQ 6 What are the causes of jaundice in pregnancy?

The causes could be:

- Medical (hepatitis, hepatotoxic drugs; hemolytic anaemia)
- Surgical jaundice (viz. gall stone)
- Icteris gravis gravidarum.
- Hepatosis of pregnancy (may be a complication of OCP, hyperemesis gravidarum, acute fatty liver, septic abortion).

SAQ 7 How will you treat malaria in pregnancy?

After confirming diagnosis of malaria by peripheral blood smear and or ELISA, the following drugs can be used for malaria.

(i) Chloroquine salts (600 mg) 4 tablets stat followed by two tablets after 6 hours, then one tablet twice daily for two days.
(ii) Alternatively amodiaquine (600 mg) 3 tablets stat; one and half tablet six hours later and one and half tablet daily for two days.
(iii) In resistant cases, pyrimethamine and sulphamethopyrazine 2 tablets stat dose and to be repeated after a week.
(iv) Quinine (600 mg) thrice daily for five days not dangerous for foetus, but may induce abortion.

SAQ 8 How will you treat toxoplasmosis in pregnancy?

Toxoplasmosis is protozoal disease caused by *Toxoplasma gondii* presents with fever and generalized lymphadenopathy, damages foetus (produces congenital anomalies, stillbirth, prematurity and abortions) diagnosed by serological methods, treated by spiramycin 250 mg 4 hourly × 10 days or sulphaphenazole 2 gm daily. Some recommends therapeutic abortion in acute maternal infection to avoid foetal damage.

SAQ 9 Name viral diseases transmitted to foetus by infected mother.

Measles, chickenpox, smallpox, influenza, rubella, poliomyelitis, hepatitis, AIDS, are transmitted to foetus from mother may lead to abortion, premature labour and congenital anomalies.

SAQ 10 How will you treat syphilis in pregnancy? What ill effect it may produce on pregnancy?

Since the *Treponema pallidum* affects the placenta and foetus producing IUFD, stillborn baby or abortion. Baby develops syphilitic lesion in infancy and childhood.

Early diagnosis of syphilis has to be made and institutional treatment with penicillin is drug of choice for pregnant woman. Procaine penicillin 4,00,000 units two vials or procaine penicillin G in aluminium stearate 2 ml 6,00,000 units for 15 days. If the patient is allergic to penicillin, erythromycin 2 gm daily in divided doses for 10 days.

SAQ 11 How will you treat gonorrhoea in pregnancy?

It is treated with procaine penicillin G 1.2 mega units of penicillin, if not treated, it may cause puerperal sepsis and ophthalmia neonatorum.

LAQ 12 What are the causes of pruritus vulvae in pregnancy?

The etiologies of pruritus vulvae in pregnancy are as follows:

Gynaecological causes	Metabolic causes	Worms	Dermatological	Physiological
• *Monilia albicans* • *Trichomonas vaginitis*	• Anaemia • Vitamin A, B deficiency • Adiposity		• Local • Generalised	Excess vaginal discharge

LAQ 13 What are the effects of diabetes mellitus on pregnancy?

These are:

Pregnancy complications

- Abortion
- Hydramnios
- Pre-eclampsia
- Maternal infection
- Premature labour
- Fall in oestrogen synthesis in facto-placental unit

Foetal effects

- IUFD
- Foetal macrosomia
- Growth retardation and delayed lung maturation
- Neonatal death
- Congenital defects

LAQ 14 Mention some hematological and biochemical changes of normal pregnancy.

The important hematological circulatory biochemical changes are as follows:

- Expansion of vascular bed and increase in oxygen consumption.
- Rise in ESR; blood volume.
- Fall in plasma proteins.
- Hydraemia causing reduction in RBC and Hb%, leukocytosis, normal platelet.

Bone marrow shows normoblastic hyperplasia. Fall in serum iron and rise in iron binding capacity. Fall in acid and pepsin in stomach.

LAQ 15 What are the complications of anaemia in pregnancy?

On mother

- Infection
- Malnutrition
- PPH
- Premature labour
- Puerperal sepsis

On foetus

- Prematurity
- More prone to neonatal death
- Stillbirth

LAQ 16 What are the indications of blood transfusion in pregnancy?

Indications of blood transfusion in pregnancy are:

- Severe anaemia seen very late.
- Anaemia not improving with haematinics.
- Aplastic anaemia, haemolytic anaemia, thrombocytopenia.
- Anaemia of infection, PPH and shock.

9 Diseases of Genital Tract in Pregnancy

SAQ 1 What are the clinical features of retroverted gravid uterus?

The clinical features of retroverted gravid uterus are as follows:

Symptoms

- No features up to 12 weeks
- Retention of urine
- Low back pain
- Constipation
- Abortion

Signs

- Retention of urine
- Cystic swelling in hypogastrium
- P/V cystic globular swelling in posterior fornix
- P/R gravid uterus in pouch of Douglas

LAQ 2 How will you treat retroverted gravid uterus?

Symptomless up to 10 weeks requires no treatment advised to lie on face twice for 15 minutes.

Continuous Foley's catheter with ampicillin and urine sensitivity, bowel evacuation.

↓

Manual reposition

↓

Hodge-Smith pessary

↓

Caesarean section if there is anterior sacculation

SAQ 3 What are effects of fibroid on pregnancy?

- Abortion
- Malpresentation
- Obstructed labour
- Uterine inertia
- Puerperal sepsis
- PPH

LAQ 4 How will you treat uterine fibroid in pregnancy?

During pregnancy

Uncomplicated

- Observation.

Complicated

- Abdominal myomectomy
- Laparotomy (for red degeneration, twisted subserous fibroid)
- Elective caesarean section.

During labour

(i) Normal delivery is expected if fibroid is not in pelvis.

(ii) Fibroid in pelvis – caesarean section with myomectomy or hysterectomy (if women over 35 years or uncontrollable PPH with living child).

SAQ 5 What effects an ovarian tumour may produce in pregnancy?

- Abdominal pain
- Dyspnoea
- Abortion
- Premature labour
- Obstructed labour
- Non-engagement
- Malpresentation

SAQ 6 How will you manage Ca cervix in pregnancy?

Ca cervix is rare (3–10,000) in pregnancy presents with irregular vaginal bleeding or blood stained white discharge, diagnosed by cervical biopsy and is treated as following:

During pregnancy

- Radical surgery with removal of early pregnancy.
- In late pregnancy caeserean section with hysterectomy.
- MTP with hysterectomy.
- MTP with radiotherapy in inoperable Ca cervix.

During labour

- Caeserean section with treatment of Ca cervix
- Spontaneous vaginal delivery with appropriate treatment of Ca cervix.

SAQ 7 What is Hingorani's sign?

When pregnant women with large ovarian cyst are placed in low head position, cystic tumour moves upwards towards epigastrium, a groove becomes visible between tumour and ovarian fundus

SAQ 8 How will you treat ovarian tumour in pregnancy?

The plan adopted as following to treat ovarian tumour in pregnancy.

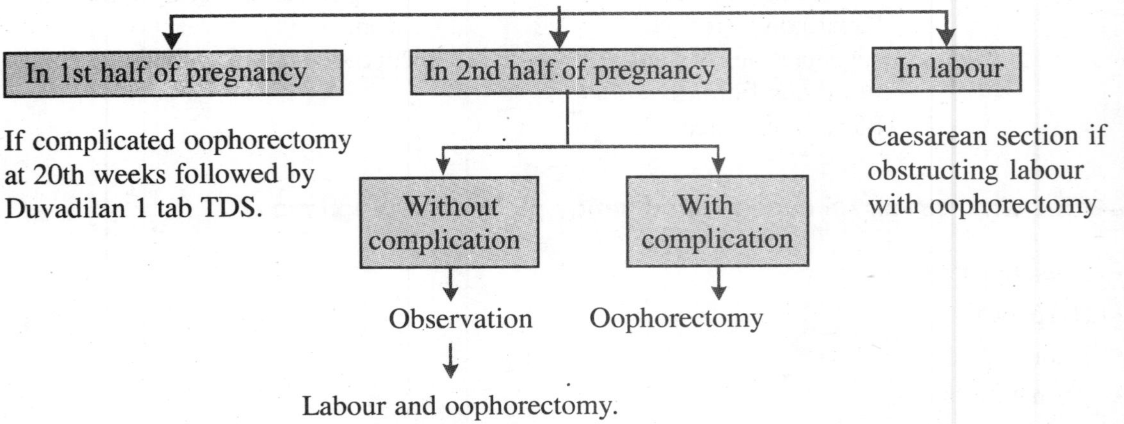

Preterm Labour; Post-term Pregnancy

10

SAQ 1 What is preterm labour?

Preterm labour is baby bore after 22nd weeks and before 37th weeks of gestation.

LAQ 2 What are the causes of preterm labour?

Maternal diseases: Anaemia, syphilis, hypertension, diabetes, toxoplasmosis, cervical incompetence, fibroid of uterus, malformation of uterus, APH, eclampsia and toxemia of pregnancy.

Foetal cause: Multiple pregnancy, Rh incompatibility, foetal malformation, hydramnios.

Iatrogenic pregnancy with IUCD; operatively terminated.

Social miscellaneous cause: Poor weight gain, small stature, smoking, overwork in domestic and outdoor.

SAQ 3 How to prevent preterm labour?

Risk factors should be corrected in antenatal check up, bed rest, hospitalization, cervical incompetence with cervical suture.

Without risk factors are given:

(i) Tocolytic agents (Isoxsuprine, beta adrenergic like salbutamol, orciprenaline, nylidrin, ritodrine, fenoterol, terbutaline).

(ii) IV infusion of 9.5% alcohol in 5% dextrose.

(iii) Prostaglandin inhibitors (indomethacin).

SAQ 4 What are the indications and contraindications of tocolytic agents in preterm labour?

Indications

- Membrane intact with mild uterine contraction

Contraindications

- Chorioamnionitis
- Fever
- Heart diseases
- APH
- Thyrotoxicosis

LAQ 5 How to manage preterm labour?

Management aims at delivery of oxygenated baby without trauma.

1st stage	2nd stage
Bed rest, avoid prolong labour if sign of foetal distress and cervix fails to progress—caesarean section.	Episiotomy; low forceps if there is delay in progress of head. Vacuum extractor is contraindicated. Baby is given suction. Oxygen, endotracheal intubation and positive pressure oxygen ventilation.

SAQ 6 What is growth retarded foetus?

Newborn baby is said to be growth retarded if birth weight falls below 10th percentile for particular gestational age or twice below standard deviation form normal values of birth weight for gestational age.

LAQ 7 What are the causes of growth retarded foetus?

The causes are as follows:

(A) **Foetal defect** (hypoplastic foetus defective organogenesis) due to chromosomal abnormalities, placental infection (syphilis, toxoplasmosis, rubella, cytomegalo).

(B) **Foetal growth defect:** Inadequate diet, anaemia, poor uteroplacental sypply (heart disease anaemia, smoking, APH, abnormal placenta, multiple pregnancy).

(C) **Others:** Genetic and racial, elderly prima or teenaged prima, hard working mother.

LAQ 8 How to detect growth retarded foetus?

It is done in following way:

1. History of risk factor, clinical examination of woman (elderly or teenaged prima), smoking habit, habitat of high altitude, PIH; malnutrition of mother, hypertension, estimation of gestational age, uterine fundus height, abdominal girth measurement at the umbilicus level.
2. Ultrasonographic examination.
3. Oestriol assay and HPL: Urinary oestriol values are lower and so is serum placental lactogen.

SAQ 9 What is post-datism/prolonged pregnancy/post-term pregnancy/postmaturity?

Prolongation of pregnancy for 14 days or beyond 40th week of pregnancy occurs in 2–10% of pregnancy called post-datism. It should be monitored for gestational age, foetal maturity and distress.

LAQ 10 How to diagnose post-datism?

This will be done in the following ways:

- History
- Clinical examination
- Radiology of foetus for ossific center of femur, tibia, thick cranial bones
- Falling level of 24 hours urinary oestriol
- Amnioscopy
- Ultrasonography
- Amniocentesis to note meconium staining creatinine level, phospholipid content, detection of fat laden aneucleated foetal cells.

SAQ 11 What are dangers of post-datism?

Big baby is difficult for labour and baby is more prone to distress.

SAQ 12 What are the signs of post-datism on delivery?

- Birth weight and length is more, not smeared by vernix caseosa
- Hard big head
- Nails beyond fingers
- Placenta showing infarction and calcification
- Meconium stained liquor amnii and scanty amnii.

SAQ 13 What is IUFD?

It is intrauterine, antepartum death of foetus after 28th weeks of pregnancy.

SAQ 14 What do you mean by: (i) spalding sign and (ii) maceration?

(i) **Spalding sign:** It is sign elicited by skiagram showing overlapping of cranial bones due to shrinkage of brain after one week of foetus death.

(ii) **Maceration:** Due to aseptic autolysis, there is cutaneous bullae formation and peeling off skin called maceration.

LAQ 15 What are the causes of IUFD?

The main causes can be classified as follows:

Diseases of pregnancy
- APH
- Pre-celampsia

Maternal diseases
- Hypertension
- Renal failure
- Syphilis
- Malaria
- Anaemia
- Drugs

Foetal causes
- Placental insufficiency
- Malformed foetus
- Rh incompatibility

LAQ 16 What are the clinical features of IUFD?

The clinical features of IUFD are as follows:

Symptoms
- Foetal movement ceases
- Dirty brown discharge P/V

Signs
- Static maternal weight and regression of signs of pregnancy
- Height of fundus less than corresponding amenorrhoea
- Foetus and uterus flaccid with no foetal movement and FHS
- Egg shell cracking of foetal head

SAQ 17 How will you diagnose IUFD?

- History
- Clinical examination
- Skiagram (spalding sign): Hyperflexon or extension of foetal spine; Gas shadows in foetal heart and vessels
- Ultrasonography and Doppler heart monitor.

SAQ 18 What complications may arise out of IUFD?

Complicatiom may be:
- Psychological upset
- Hypofibrinogenaemia

- Absorption of toxic products from dead foetus
- PPH
- Uterine inertia

SAQ 19 How to treat IUFD?

- Uterus generally expels the dead foetus within 2 weeks,
- Induction of labour by syntocinon or prostaglandins,
- Fresh blood transfusion for haemorrhagic conditions.

SAQ 20 Why intra-amniotic hypertonic saline or low amniotomy are not recommended for induction of labour in case of IUFD?

Intra-amniotic hypertonic saline produces hypernatraemia and coagulopathy may occur and low amniotomy produces infection, therefore, these are not recommended method of induction of labour in IUFD.

11 Normal Labour

SAQ 1 Define normal labour or eutocia.

The process of expulsion of mature foetus, presented by vertex per vagina followed by expulsion of after birth where parturition is uncomplicated, spontaneous and not delayed. Abnormal labour is called dystocia. The first pregnancy for labour is called primigravida and subsequent pregnancy at labour is called multipara.

SAQ 2 What factors initiate labour?

Factors initiating labour are:

(i) Uterine distension

(ii) Hormones: (a) Progesterone block, (b) oestrogen, (c) prostaglandin synthesis, (d) uterine sensitivity of oxytocin

(iii) α adrenergic response

(iv) Foetal pituitary adrenal activity

SAQ 3 What are stages of normal labour?

It has following arbitrarily stages:

1st stage	2nd stage	3rd stage
Cervical dilatation stage. For primi, it is 10 hours and for multigravida 5 hours.	Stage of delivery of foetus. It is 1 hour and ½ hour for primi- and multigravida, respectively.	Up to expulsion of placenta, umbilical cord and membranes. It is about 5 minutes for both multi- and primigravida.

SAQ 4 What do you mean by fundal dominance and uterine pacemaker?

In normal uterus, the strength and duration of contraction is maximum in fundus called fundal dominance and uterine contraction in labour originate near uterine end of one of the fallopian tube called uterine pacemaker.

SAQ 5 What pressure change occurs in uterus in labour?

Resting intrauterine pressure in first stage in between contraction is 5–8 mm Hg and its intensity increases to 40–60 mm Hg. In second stage, the same are 10 mm Hg and raises to 110 mm Hg. Pain is felt when pressure raises to 25 mm Hg.

SAQ 6 What do you mean by caul?

When cervix is fully dilated, the forewater usually ruptures and head plugs the cervical canal with afterwater. When chorion ruptures and foetal head is delivered with covering of amnion; then baby is said to born in caul.

SAQ 7 What do you mean by effacement of cervix?

Effacement of cervix means progressive merging of cervical canal with hemispherical lower uterine segment clinically detected by obliteration of cervical canal.

SAQ 8 Describe the following terminologies: (a) Sagittal suture, (b) Frontal suture, (c) Coronal suture, (d) Lambdoidal suture, (e) Bregma, (f) Lambda.

(a) **Sagittal suture:** It lies in midline across the vault of the skull.

(b) **Frontal suture:** It is in between two halves of frontal bone.

(c) **Coronal suture:** Frontal and parietal bones are separated by coronal suture.

(d) **Lambdoidal suture:** It separates parietal from occipital bones.

(e) **Bregma** (anterior fontanel): Unossified membrane with angles continuous with frontal, sagittal, right and left coronal sutures.

(f) **Lambda** (posterior fontanel): It is triangular depression at junction of sagittal and lambdoidal sutures.

LAQ 9 How the true pelvis is bounded?

It is bounded as follows:

Inlet	Cavity	Outlet
Bounded by upper border of symphysis pubis, pubic crest, iliopectineal line, sacroiliac joint and sacral promontory from before backward. **True conjugate**: Sacral promontory to mid-point of upper border of symphysis pubis (10–8 cm or 4¼".) **Obstetric conjugate**: Centre of sacral promontory to nearest mid-point upon posterior-surface of symphysis pubis (10 cm 4".) **Transverse diameter** 5¼" (13.2 cm) distance between furthest apart points on ilio-pectineal line joining the midpoint between iliopectineal eminence and sacroiliac joint. **Oblique diameter** 4¾" (12 cm) distance between one sacroiliac joint to opposite ilio-pectineal eminence.	Bounded above by plane of inlet and below by plane of outlet, anteriorly by symphysis pubis and posteriorly by sacrum and coccyx. Its anteroposterior diameter: Transverse diameter and oblique diameter is 4¾" (12 cm); therefore its plane is rounded.	Bounded by lower border of symphysis pubis, laterally by ischeal spines and posteriorly by the tip of the sacrum. Anteroposterior diameter extending inferior border of symphysis pubis to tip of sacrum $4^1/_4$" (13.2 cm), transverse $4^1/_5$" (10.5 cm) diameter and oblique diameter is 4¾" (12 cm).

SAQ 10 What is curve of carus?

Curve of carus or anatomical pelvic axis is curved line with concavity forward, obtained by joining the axis of the true pelvis.

SAQ 11 How the false pelvis is bounded?

It is bounded anteriorly by abdominal wall posteriorly by lumbar vertebrae and laterally by iliac fossae.

SAQ 12 Describe the following regions of foetal skull: (a) Vertex, (b) Brow, (c) Face, (d) Sinciput, (e) Occiput.

(a) **Vertex** of foetal skull is bounded by anterior fontanel and coronal suture anteriorly and lambdoid suture and posterior fontanel posteriorly, commonly presented in labour.
(b) **Brow:** It is the area from root of the nose and supraorbital ridges to anterior fontanel and coronal sutures.

(c) **Face** is the area from root of nose, supraorbital ridges to the floor of the mouth.
(d) **Sinciput**: Midpoint region of the forehead.
(e) **Occiput**: External occipital protuberance.

SAQ 13 What do you mean by the following presentation—
(a) Vertex, (b) Brow, (c) Face?

Vertex	Brow	Face
It is fully flexed suboccipito-bregmatic circumference passing true pelvis.	Partially flexed mentovertical circumference passing true pelvis.	Extended submento-bregmatic circumfere-nce passing true pelvis.

SAQ 14 Define the following terminologies—
(a) Lie, (b) Attitude, (c) Presentation and presenting parts, (d) Denominator, (e) Position, (f) Engagement.

(a) **Lie:** Relation of long axis of foetus with mother, viz. longitudinal, transverse, oblique.

(b) **Attitude:** Relation of different parts of foetus with each other is called attitude, viz. flexion, deflexion, extension.

(c) **Presentation and presenting parts:** It is the part of the foetus presents at lower pole of uterus, presenting part enters the pelvis.

(d) **Denominator:** It is the arbitrarily fixed point of any presentation coming in relation to different quadrants in pelvis.

(e) **Position:** The relation of denominator to different quadrants of pelvis, viz. LOA; ROA, etc.

(f) **Engagement:** When the maximum transverse diameter of any presentation passes pelvic brim.

SAQ 15 What are the reasons of head presentation?

(i) Due to gravity

(ii) Due to better accumulation of broad breech at fundus and smaller head below.

SAQ 16 What comes out in 3rd stage of labour?

Placenta, membranes and cord.

SAQ 17 How the placenta are separated?

By bearing down efforts or by obstetrician by at Schultz method or Duncan method.

SAQ 18 Define mechanism of normal labour.

It is the series of movements by foetus at birth passage during expulsion in normal labour.

SAQ 19 What are the steps of movement in normal labour?

Engagement
↓
Descent and flexion
↓
Internal rotation
↓
Extension of head
↓
Restitution
↓
External rotation
↓
Lateral flexion

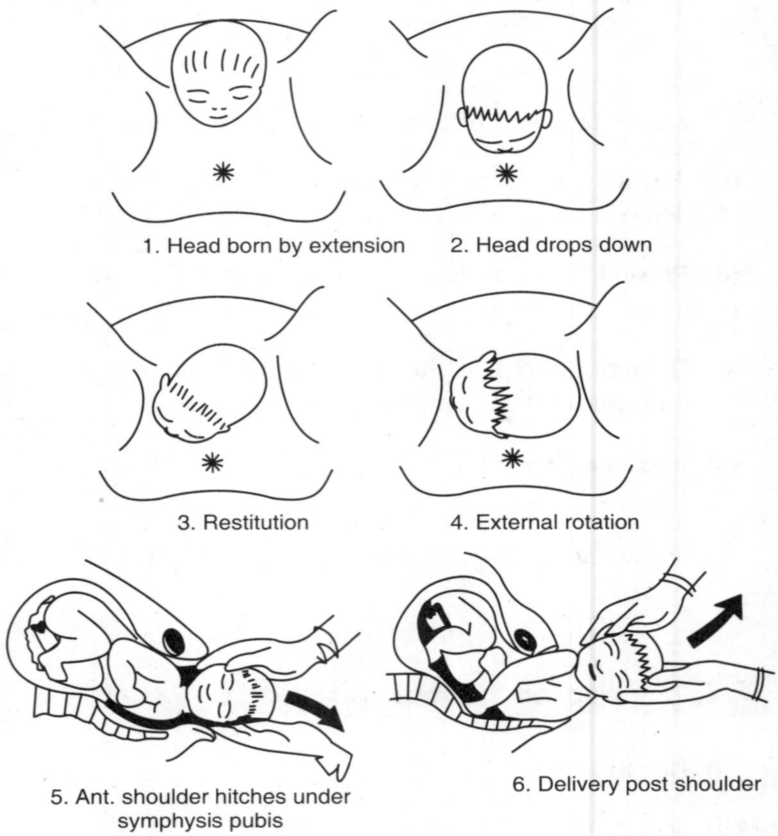

SAQ 20 Define: (a) moulding of head, (b) caput succedaneum.

(a) Moulding of head: This is one of the effect of labour, when there is alteration in the shape of foetal head and reduction in its size produced by resistance in birth passage during labour. It is physiological, helps easy passage of head in birth canal and is harmless.

(b) Caput succedaneum: Due to interference of venous and lymphatic drainage of area by pressure of dilating cervix, vagina, there is localized oedema of foetal scalp occurs during labour called caput succedaneum.

SAQ 21 What are the differences between true and false pain of labour?

These are:

True pain	False pain
• Pain	• Non-progressive and non-rhythmical
• Show	• No bag of forewater
• Hardening of uterus	• Cervix not dilated,
• Progressive dilatation of cervix.	• Pain may be relieved by enema.
• Bag of forewater	

SAQ 22 What are the phases of Friedman partograph?

When cervical dilatation against labour is plotted by Friedman, it shows the following phases.

(i) Latent phase (variable duration).

(ii) Phase of acceleration, cervix 2–3 cm dilated.

(iii) Phase of deceleration when cervix is fully dilated.

SAQ 23 What is show?

It is discharge of blood-stained mucus due to expulsion of cervical mucus plug and blood from separated membranes from lower uterine segment. It is a sign of 1st stage of labour.

LAQ 24 What are the clinical features of normal labour?

These are as follows:

1st stage

Symptom

(i) Pain.
(ii) Show. (Discharge of blood-stained mucus P/V)

Signs

(i) Rise of BP and temperature.
(ii) Hardening of uterus.
(iii) Progressive dilatation of cervical canal and show.

2nd stage

Symptom

(i) Bag of forewater.
(ii) Bearing down pain and desire to pass stool.

Signs

(i) Hardening of uterus.
(ii) FHS position descents.
(iii) Anus gaps.
(iv) Hairy head are visualized

3rd stage

Symptom

(i) Shivering of body.

Signs

(i) Pt.relaxing.
(ii) Gush of liquor amnii is discharged.
(iii) Uterus firm not moving side by side
(iv) After placental separation, uterus globular and more mobile side by side.
(v) Cord descends outside vagina.
(vi) Placental delivery followed by vaginal discharge of clot about 100-200 ml blood.

LAQ 25 What are the types of normal labour?

The normal labour is of three types.

Spontaneous active labour

It starts spontaneously and completes actively within 12 hours and 6 hours in primi- and multigravida, respectively.

Accelerated active labour

Inactive labour activated by low rupture of membrane oxytocin drip, in 1st and 2nd stage

Induced active labour

Labour induced by LRM or oxytocin drip

SAQ 26 What are the signs and symptoms of maternal and foetal distress in prolong labour?

They are as follows:

Maternal distress	Foetal distress
• Exhausted facing • Dehydrated tongue • Pulse more than 100/m • Protein and acetone in urine.	• FHS more than 160 or less than 120 with irregularity • Excess foetal movement • Meconium P/V. • Faetal acidaemia, more caput on vertex.

SAQ 27 What is the principle of management of 2nd stage of labour?

Birth of non-asphyxiated baby in aseptic condition without damaging perineum.

SAQ 28 How to protect perineum from injury in 2nd stage of labour?

(i) By preventing rapid progress of head in violent pains and maintaining flexion of head.
(ii) Liberal episiotomy if there is threatening of tear to perineum.
(iii) Guarding the head and shoulders during the delivery.

SAQ 29 What could be the reason, if head is born with no further progress?

(i) Cord round neck
(ii) Oblique position of the shoulders. Here head should be depressed between two palms towards perineum till anterior shoulder brought under symphysis pubis. Fundal pressure and traction on head by palm. In the next step, head is lifted towards mothers abdomen, so that posterior shoulder can be delivered followed by anterior shoulder delivery.

LAQ 30 How to manage the first stage of labour?

Broadly, the steps of management are as follows:

(i) General examination with obstetrical examination to see cephalopelvic disproportion, FHS
(ii) Evacuation of bladder and bowel.
(iii) Aseptic dressing.
(iv) Relief of pain
(v) Only water orally
(vi) Foetal status and maternal vital sign monitoring during labour.
(vii) Partography ascending for cervical dilatation and descending for foetal head descend.

SAQ 31 What equipment should be kept ready for home delivery?

Following apparatus should be kept ready before home delivery—Catheter, enema apparatus, sponge holding forceps, scissors, dissecting forceps, needles, needle holder, Kocher's artery forceps, sutures, mucus catheter, kidney dish, bowl, obstetric forceps, rubber sheets, gloves, gown, cord ligatures, masks, surgical dressings, drugs like pethidine, sparine, ergometrine, syntocinon, lethidrone, spirit, local anaesthetics.

SAQ 32 What are the signs of placental separation?

They are as follows:

1. Uterus in hard, globular mobile side to side.
2. Fundus rises above the level of delivery.
3. Permanent lengthening of the cord outside vulva.
4. If by gentle pressure uterus is drawn up and by doing this if cord at vulva is drawn up, then placenta is unseparated.

SAQ 33 What are the different methods to deliver placenta?

These are:

Fundal pressure	Brandt-Andrews method
After placenta is separated, it is delivered by bearing down pain.	Here uterus is pushed gently upwards and cord is pulled out, taking the precaution of not inverting the uterus, i.e. controlled cord traction.

SAQ 34 What are the points to be noticed after delivery of the baby?

The points to be noticed are as follows:

(i) Baby's respiratory passage should be clear.
(ii) Note birth time, weight, height, sex, identification marks.
(iii) Note congenital defects.
(iv) By olive oil and cotton swab vernix is removed, soap water bath is given.
(v) Antiseptic dressing applied on stump.

Complications of Third Stage Labour

12

SAQ 1 Mention the important complications of third stage of labour.

- Retained placenta
- PPH
- Shock
- Sepsis
- Inversion of uterus
- Embolism (thrombus, air)

SAQ 2 What are the causes of retained placenta?

- Atonic uterus
- Constriction ring
- Morbid adhesion of placenta

SAQ 3 What is PPH?

It is excessive haemorrhage from genital tract after birth up to end of puerperium. It may be third stage haemorrhage; haemorrhage within 24 hours, i.e. primary PPH or puerperal haemorrhage 24 hours after delivery, i.e. secondary PPH.

SAQ 4 What are the different dangers of PPH?

- Shock
- Sepsis
- Lactation may fail
- Anaemia
- Embolism
- Thrombophlebitis
- Sheehan's syndrome

SAQ 5 What are the different methods to remove retained placenta?

(i) Credes expression method by squeezing uterus per abdomen.

(ii) Patient put on lithotomy position and under GA hand is inserted in uterus along cleavage plane of the placenta. Left hand steadies uterus per abdomen and placenta is removed the method is called manual removal of placenta.

(iii) Hysterectomy.

SAQ 6 What are the causes of secondary postpartum haemorrhage?

- Retained placenta or membrane
- Blood clots
- Caesarean section wound/subinvolution
- Injury to cervix

SAQ 7 What are the different causes of shock in obstetrics practice?

It may be:

1. Haemorrhagic
2. Non-haemorrhagic
   (a) Trauma of obstetric procedure
   (b) Prolonged labour
   (c) Toxaemia
   (d) Anaesthetics
   (e) Mendelson's syndrome
   (f) Embolism
   (g) Neurogenic
   (h) Endotoxic shock

SAQ 8 What is inversion of uterus?

It is turning inside out of uterus when fundus reaches internal os it is 1st degrees, when fundus reaches external os and uterus up to internal os it is said to be 2nd degree and when uterus and cervix is completely inverted it is 3rd degree with fundus protruding out of vaginal introitus.

LAQ 9 What are the clinical features of inversion of uterus?

They are:

Symptoms

- Shock or vaginal bleeding,
- Something coming down P/V
- Pelvic pain and difficulty in micturition.

Signs

- Shows cupping up of uterus
- Fundus cannot be felt
- Protrusion of fundus outside uterus.

LAQ 10 How to treat inversion of uterus?

Prophylaxis: Avoid Crede's method and unnecessary manipulation of uterus—Push uterus inside under GA in recent cases. If inversion occurs after few days then uterus is pushed with aseptic vaginal douche called O'sullivain's hydrostatic method. Subacute inversion due to delay is treated with Aveiling repositor, chronic inversion is treated operatively by Haultain's method per abdominally or Spinelli's method per vaginally.

13

Abnormal Presentation

SAQ 1 What is occipitoposterior position of vertex?

This is vertex presentation with occiput lying, either against right or left sacroiliac joint, the reason being android or anthropoid pelvis, deflexed head or large foetus or uterine inertia.

LAQ 2 How to diagnose occipitoposterior position?

Inspection	Palpation	Auscultation	P/V	Radiology
Flat supra-pubic region	Breech in fundal grip limbs in front, delay in engagement.	FHS heard on flank.	Elongated bag of membranes; sagittal suture obliquely placed; posterior fontanel near sacroiliac joint.	Confirms diagnosis, station and degree of flexion, type of pelvis.

SAQ 3 What types of course occur in occipitoposterior position?

There may be:

(i) Delay in labour

(ii) Spontaneous or assisted vaginal delivery

(iii) Arrest of malrotated head with its ill effect.

SAQ 4 What is deep transverse arrest?

In case of mild deflection of head in occipitoposterior position, occiput rotates 1/8 circle anteriorly while reaching pelvic floor and both occiput and sinciput comes under pubic arch causing arrest of head in transverse diameter called deep transverse arrest.

LAQ 5 What is the mechanism of labour of occipitoposterior position of vertex?

1. Engagement in occipitoposterior position.

↓

2. Descent.

- **With flexion of head**

  Long internal rotation of occiput and comes under pubic arch, with rotation of shoulder at right angle.

  ↓

  Extension.

  ↓

  Restitution.

  ↓

  External rotation.

  ↓

  Lateral flexion.

- **Without complete flexion of head**

  Generally there is arrest on pelvic floor depending upon deflexion, uterine inertia and pelvic types.

  ↓

  - **Mild deflexion**

    Occiput rotates $^1/_8$ circle anterior and sinciput and occiput reaches pelvic floor both sinciput and occiput come under pubic arch causing transversely arrest of head in pelvis called deep transverse arrest.

  - **Moderate deflexion**

    Occiput and sinciput touches pelvic floor at the same time causing oblique occipitoposterior arrest.

  - **Extreme deflexion**

    Sinciput touches and rotates 1/8 circle to come under pubic arch and occiput comes under sacrum persistent occiput posterior

    ↓

    Face to pubis possible with small head pushed down nose, pubic arch, vertex and occiput born by flexion and face by extension

SAQ 6 What is oblique occipitoposterior arrest?

In case of moderate deflection of head in occipitoposterior position of head sinciput and occiput touches in same time in oblique diameter of pelvis with occipitoposterior called oblique occipitoposterior arrest.

SAQ 7 What is persistant occipitoposterior or occipitosacral arrest?

In case of extreme deflection in occipitoposterior position, sinciput touches the pelvic floor first and makes 1/8th circle rotation to come under pubic arch and occiput comes in the hollow of the sacrum called persistant occipitoposterior or occipitosacral arrest.

SAQ 8 What points should be observed in P/V examination in case of occipitoposterior postion?

(i) Cervical dilatation
(ii) Position of arrest in occiput, attitude, station of foetal head
(iii) Pelvic assessment
(iv) Caput formation.

SAQ 9 How to deliver with engaged head with full dilatation, adequate pelvic capacity and with deep transverse arrest and oblique occipitoposterior arrest?

Quick manual rotation of head with mid forceps delivery under local or general anaesthesia in a septic condition and emptying urinary bladder.

SAQ 10 How to deliver occipitosacral arrest of occipitoposterior position?

After episiotomy, mid forceps delivery of baby is done from face to pubis in primigravida. It occurs in anthropoid pelvis. Higher head arrest requires manual rotation, followed by forceps delivery.

SAQ 11 What are the different positions of face presentation?

These are RMP; LMP; LMA; RMA.

SAQ 12 When to opt for Kielland forceps, vacuum extractor, caesarean forceps, craniotomy?

Kielland forceps: It is done in occipitosacral arrest where instead of manual rotation Kielland forceps rotation and delivery is done.

Vacuum extractor: If there is thin cervical rim.

Caesarean section: When there is uterine inertia and cervical dilatation.

Craniotomy: Dead foetus head is impacted in pelvis in OP position.

SAQ 13 What is face presentation?

Face presents when head is in attitude of extension comprises mouth with alveolar margin nose, eyes, mentum, malar eminences.

SAQ 14 What are causes of face presentation?

- Contracted pelvis
- Congenital malformation (goiter, cord round neck, anencephalus, long foetal head, abnormal extension tone of neck muscle)
- Large foetus.

LAQ 15 How to diagnose face presentation?

Diagnostic points are:

Per abdomen

Fundal grip shows breech.
Lateral grip mentoanterior limbs in front, mentoposterior back in front.
Pelvic grip – head is bulkier with delayed engagement.
FHS (mentoanterior) – audible in spino-umbilical line.
Mentoposterior on flanks.

Per vagina

Elongated bag of membranes, foetal mouth, nose, eyes, alveolar margins can be palpated.

SAQ 16 When to go for forceps delivery in face presentation?

Forceps delivery in face presentation is indicated when cervix is fully dilated with adequate pelvis and presenting part arrested in pelvic cavity, manual rotation of face and trunk should be done before hand vaginally.

SAQ 17 When caesarean section is performed for face presentation?

- Uterine inertia
- Prolapse of cord
- Large baby
- Posterior face presentation.

SAQ 18 When to go for craniotomy in face presentation?

Uncared, impacted dead foetus with mentoposterior face presentation.

SAQ 19 What are the steps in mechanism of face presentation?

Following steps of mechanism occur in face presentation the event differ for position of LMA; RMP; LMP.

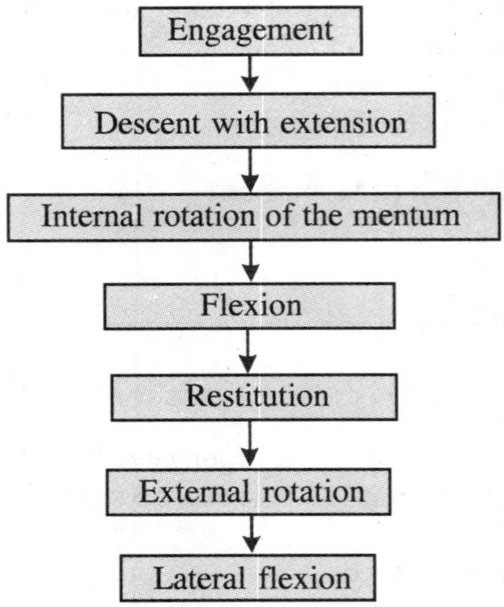

SAQ 20 What could be the different course of labour in face presentation?

- Delayed labour
- Perineal tears
- Premature rupture of membranes
- Third stage complications, viz. PPH.

SAQ 21 What is brow presentation?

Brow presentation occurs when head lies between full extension and flexion.

SAQ 22 How to diagnose brow presentation?

Diagnosis is often missed. P/V shows supraorbital ridges, anterior fontanel, smooth forehead.

SAQ 23 What are the different positions of brow presentation?

These are mentoanterior and mentoposterior brow.

SAQ 24 What is shoulder presentation?

When long axis of foetus lying transversely or obliquely across the uterus, it presents with shoulder and presenting part consists of acromion process, axilla upper part of chest wall and scapula. Rarely chest or abdomen may present instead of shoulder. Prolapse of an arm is common.

SAQ 25 What are the different positions in shoulder presentation?

These are dorsoanterior (right or left); dorsoposterior (right or left) occasionally dorsosuperior or dorsoinferior.

SAQ 26 What are the causes of shoulder presentation?

- Lax uterus
- Pelvic contraction
- Placenta praevia
- Malformed uterus
- Pelvic tumour
- Prematurity
- Twins
- Hydramnios
- Hydrocephalus

LAQ 27 How to diagnose a shoulder presentation?

Per abdomen

Inspection:
Abdomen vertically short and transversely long.
Lateral grip breech and head found in opposite side
FHS: Heard below umbilicus.

Per vagina

After rupture of long elongated membrane, upper part of arm, axilla, ribs of chest, prolapsed arm may be felt. Radiology confirms diagnosis and pelvis.

SAQ 28 How the shoulder presented foetus are borne?

Favourable termination

- Spontaneous correction of lie.
- Spontaneous version to breech.
- Spontaneous evolution and expulsion.

Unfavourable termination

- Impacted shoulder.
- Early rupture of membranes with uterine inertia

SAQ 29 What are the contraindication of external cephalic version in case of shoulder presentation?

It is done after 32 weeks of pregnancy if there is no contracted pelvis, placenta previa, uterine deformity.

SAQ 30 What is the contraindication of internal podalic version?

It is done when foetus is alive with or without hand prolapse, uterus contracts and relaxes, under general anaesthesia generally in 2nd twin baby if the uterus is not retracted.

SAQ 31 When decapitation and evisceration is done in transverse lie?

These are destructive operation performed in shoulder presentation in the following conditions.

Decapitation	Evisceration
FHS absent, head is accessible from vagina.	FHS absent, no space for decapitation.

SAQ 32 What are the complications of internal podalic version?

- Rupture uterus
- Puerperal sepsis
- Shock
- Foetal death
- Third stage complications

SAQ 33 What is unstable lie?

The different changing lie and presentation during pregnancy is called unstable lie.

SAQ 34 What are the causes of unstable lie?

- Placenta previa
- CPD
- Pelvic tumour
- Hydramnios malformation of uterus
- Hydrocephalus
- Grandmultipara with pendulous abdomen.

SAQ 35 What is breech presentation?

Here the foetal lie is longitudinal with presentation of podalic extremities comprising buttocks with lower limbs, knee or foot.

SAQ 36 What are the different types of breech?

- Complete flexed breech
- Incomplete breech
- Frank breech with extended legs and thighs flexed
- Extended thighs with either knee presentation or footling presentation.

SAQ 37 What are the different positions in breech?

Here sacrum is the denominator and the different positions could be:

- Left sacroanterior
- Right sacroanterior
- Left sacroposterior
- Right sacroposterior.

SAQ 38 What are the causes of breech?

Before 32 weeks, breech is common. The causes of breech at term are:

- Prematurity
- Twins
- Hydrocephalus
- Extended legs
- Contracted pelvis
- Placenta praevia
- Oligohydramnios
- Hydramnios
- Lack of uterine tone

LAQ 39 How to diagnose breech presentation?

Per abdomen

Fundal grip—head can be felt.
Lateral grip—limbs and back on either side.
Pelvic grip—broad breech.
FHS at higher level.

Per vagina

- During pregnancy: Absence of suture.
- During labour: After rupture of membrane, ischeal tuberosities, sacrum, spine, genitals, anus can be palpated.

Radiography

Confirms types of breech, foetal abnormalities, pelvic defects and types.

LAQ 40 Describe the mechanism of delivery of breech.

There are three deliveries occur in breech: (i) Breech, (ii) shoulder, (iii) after coming head.

Breech sacroanterior → **Shoulder** → **Head**

Breech sacroanterior

Engagement in LSA in bitroch-anteric diameter.
↓
Descent of buttocks in pelvic cavity.
↓
Internal rotation of anterior buttock, occiput 1/8th of the circle to come under pubic arch.
↓
Lateral flexion of buttocks posterior buttocks comes first then anterior
Trunk comes out by flexion.

Shoulder

Engagement of shoulder in bis-acromial diameter.
↓
Internal rotation of anterior $^{1}/_{8}$ of circle.
↓
Restitution of anterior shoulder.
↓
External rotation of the shoulder making foetus dorsoanterior.

Head

Engagement occurs in suboccipitobregmatic or suboccipitofrontal diameter
↓
Descent and flexion.
↓
Internal rotation of occiput $^{1}/_{8}$th of circle and suboccipt comes under public arch
↓
Head born in full flexion

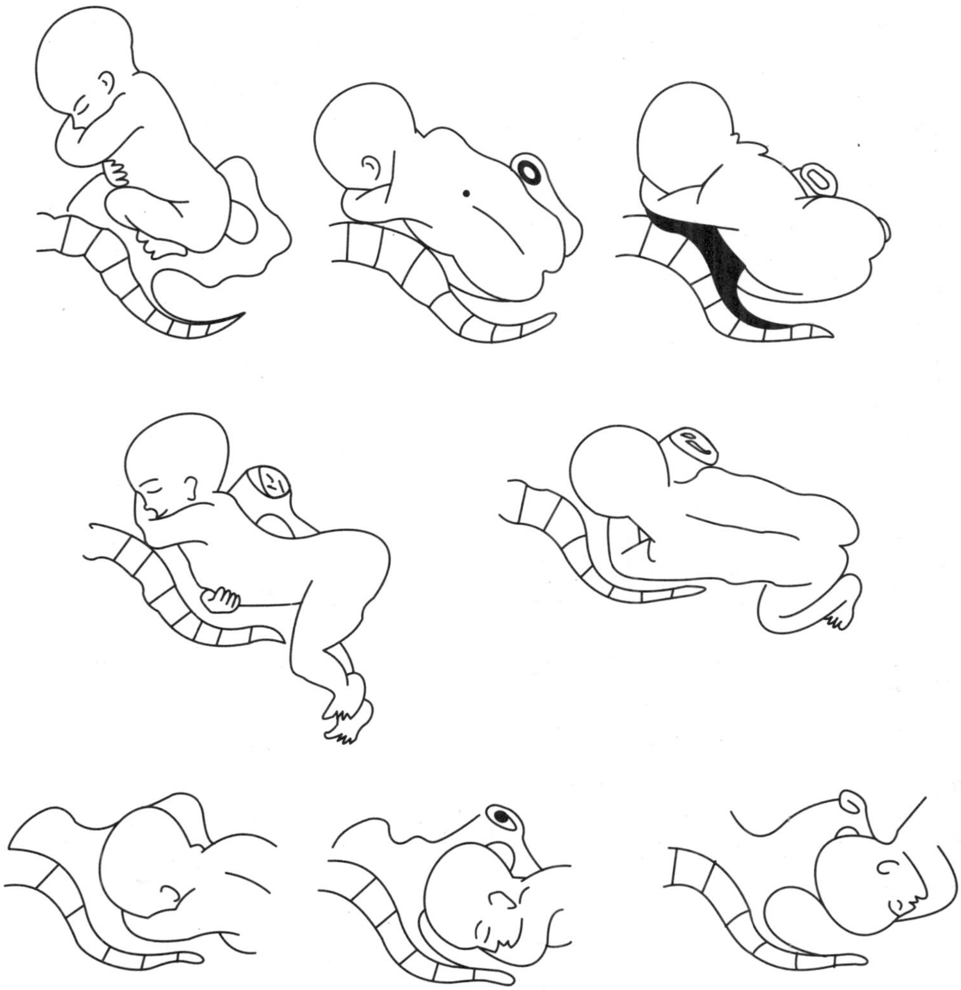

SAQ 41 What are the different foetal risks in breech presentation?

- Intracranial injury
- Prematurity
- Injuries to soft parts, dislocation of joints.

SAQ 42 When to go for external cephalic version in breech?

After 32 weeks, generally at 34 to 36 weeks.

SAQ 43 What are contraindication of external cephalic version?

- Twin pregnancy
- IUGR
- Placenta praevia
- Hypertension and toxaemia
- Elderly primi
- Previous caesarean section
- Malformation
- IUFD
- Contracted pelvis

SAQ 44 What are the dangers of external cephalic version?

External cephalic version should be done by expert obstetrician where facilities for breech delivery is there. It runs the following risks:

(i) Premature placental separation and APH

(ii) Premature labour onset

(iii) Presentation of cord and looping of cord around foetus

(iv) Presentation of footling and head.

SAQ 45 What are the indications of caesarean section in breech presentation?

Elective caesarean section is done in:

(i) Primigravida with big baby

(ii) Growth retarded foetus

(iii) Contracted pelvis.

SAQ 46 When to apply forceps for head delivery in breech?

Das's forceps are applied if head delivery is lying in pelvic cavity and does not come spontaneously.

LAQ 47 What are favourable for vaginal and caesarean section for breech?

Favourable for vaginal in breech	Favourable for caesarean section in breech
(i) Gestational age 38–41weeks with estimated foetal weight 2.5–3 kg.	(i) Gestational age below 37 or above 41 weeks, foetal weight more than 3 kg.
(ii) Cervix soft dilated	(ii) Presenting part above 1 station.
(iii) Large pelvis	(iii) Cervix firm
(iv) Earlier breech delivery	(iv) Small pelvis
(v) No maternal risk	(v) Inefficient uterine contraction
(vi) Active uterine contraction	(vi) Rupture of membrane early
(vii) Presenting part below station.	(vii) Maternal risk factors like elderly primi, hypertension diabetes
	(viii) History of difficult vaginal delivery.

SAQ 48 When to give groin traction in breech?

It is applied for breech with extended legs. If groin traction fails in dead impacted breech, breech hook can be applied.

SAQ 49 What are the causes of arrest of buttocks of foetus in pelvic cavity?

(i) Contracted pelvis, (ii) weak uterine contractions, (iii) big baby, (iv) extended legs.

SAQ 50 What is Lovset method?

It is the safest method for delivering extended arm in breech presentation where posterior shoulder below sacral promontory is rotated forwards to come under symphysis pubis and anterior arm is delivered. The other shoulder is rotated reversely for delivery.

IAQ 51 What is Burns-Marshal method?

It is assisted breech delivery for delivery of after coming head where mother lies in lithotomy position, baby is allowed to hang by its own weight unsupported for about a minute, when suboccipital area (hair margin) is seen, baby is lifted towards mothers abdomen catching baby's leg above ankle generally helpful in average size baby in multigravida.

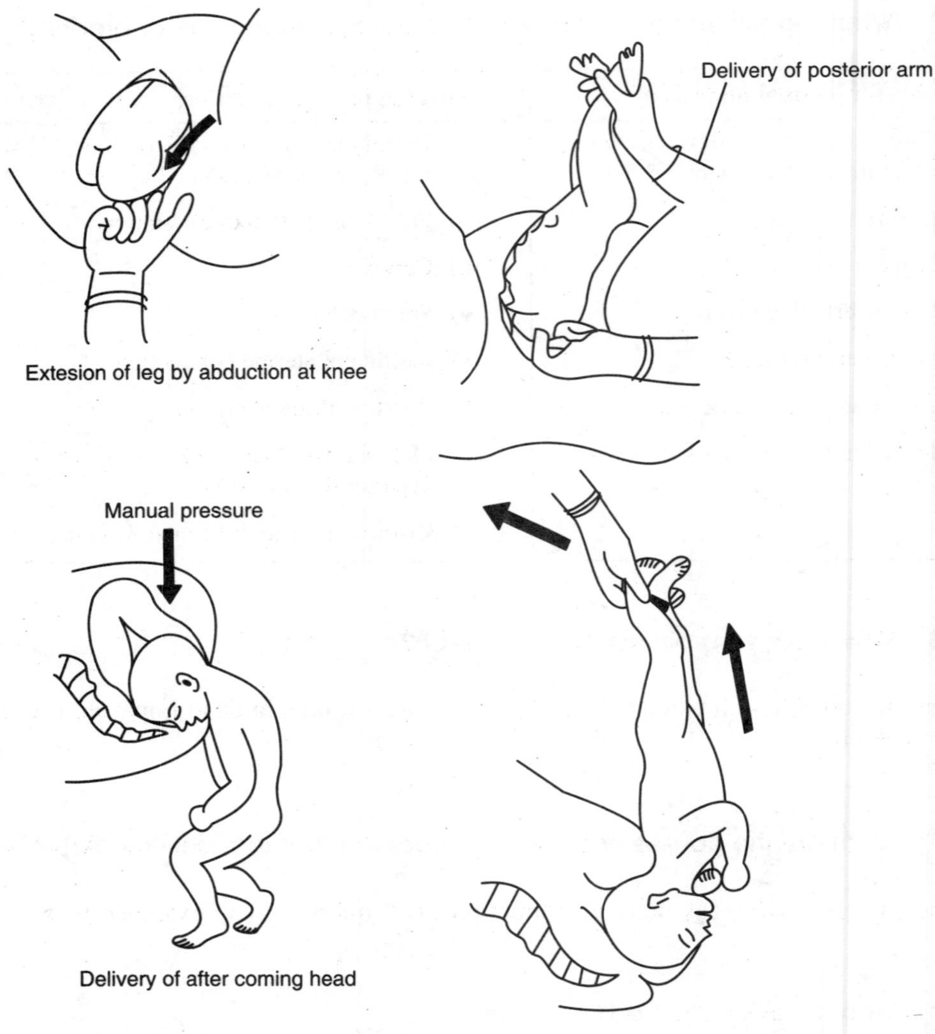

Burns-Marshal method

SAQ 52 What is breech extraction?

Under GA breech is delivered quickly for foetal distress, prolapse of cord, second twin baby in second stage of labour called breech extraction.

SAQ 53 What are causes of delay of aftercoming head in breech?

- Deflexed head
- Pelvic contraction and rigid perineum

- Undilated cervix
- Occipitoposterior
- Hydrocephalus

SAQ 54 When to go for jaw flexion, shoulder traction?

Done under GA; foetus body lie astride of obstetricians left arm. Left index and middle finger placed on molar prominence for jaw flexion. Right index and ring finger are forked on shoulder from behind. Foetus is pulled down and back till nape comes under pubic arch then towards mothers abdomen. Assistant gives suprapubic pressure to deliver the head.

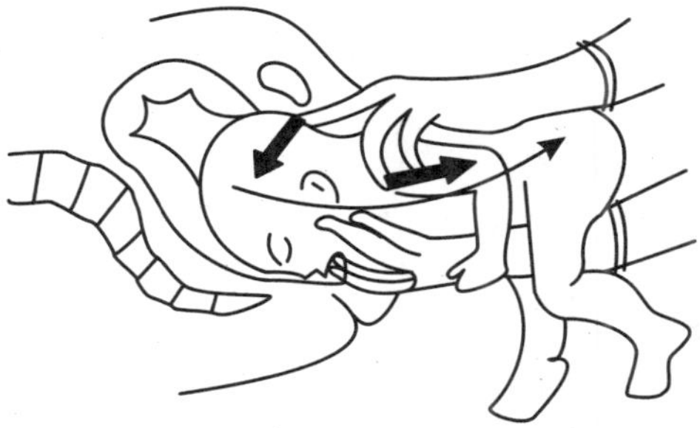

Jaw flexion and shoulder traction

SAQ 55 What is spontaneous breech delivery?

A small number of breech delivers spontaneously, where baby is only supported on birth. It is soldom with mature baby.

14 Multiple Pregnancy: Hydramnios

SAQ 1 What is multiple pregnancy?

Development of more than one foetus in pregnant uterus, may be monozygotic or dizygotic.

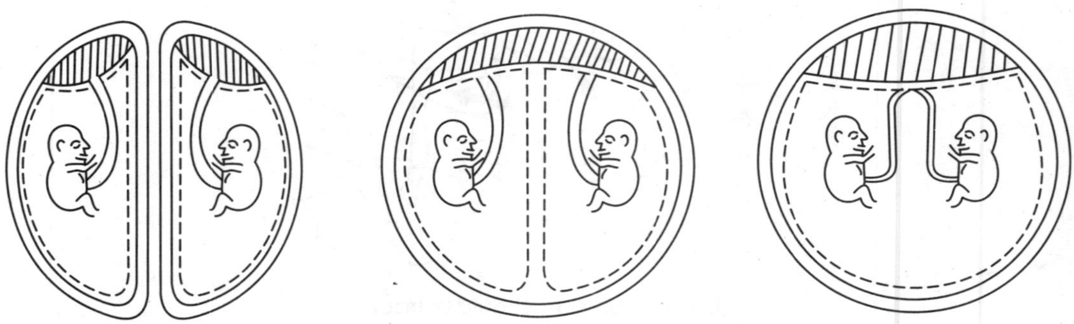

SAQ 2 What are the characteristic of mono- or dizygotic multiple pregnancy?

Monozygotic	Dizygotic
• Occurs due to early division of single fertilized ovum.	• Two ova are fertilized.
• Same sex and blood group.	• Sex may vary.
• Timing of division determines number of placenta, amnion or chorion.	• Two placenta, amnion and chorion.

SAQ 3 What are the causes of dizygotic twins?

Race, heridity, maternal age and parity, ovulation inducing agent are probable reason for it.

SAQ 4 What are the clinical features of twin pregnancy?

Symptoms

- Symptoms of cardiorespiratory distress
- Oedema
- Insomnia
- PET

Signs

- Large abdomen
- Fundus height enlarged
- Two small heads
- Two FHS
- P/V may give evidence of twins

Investigations

- Radiology
- USG

SAQ 5 What is twin transfusion syndrome?

In monozygotic twins, one baby may bleed in second one, there is generally difference of Hb by 5 gm, so one baby is anaemic and other plethoric called twin transfusion syndrome. The blood of plethoric baby has to be let down to prevent cardial failure.

LAQ 6 What are the complications of twin pregnancy?

Complications in pregnancy

- Premature onset
- PET
- Hydramnios
- Anaemia
- Placenta praevia
- Malpresentation or formation
- Foetus papyraceus or compresses

Complications in labour

- Early membrane rupture
- Prolongation of 2nd stage
- Malpresentation and locking
- 3rd stage complication PPH; retained placenta

SAQ 7 What are the different methods of managing locked twins?

Depending upon situation, it is managed by:

(i) Disengagement under anesthesia for assisted vaginal delivery
(ii) Sacrificing first baby
(iii) Caesarean section.

SAQ 8 What is superfoetation and superfecundation?

Superfoetation	Superfecundation
Fertilization of second ovum who is already pregnant.	It means fertilization of two ova which have been discharged from ovary at the same period and fertilized by two separate act of coitus.

SAQ 9 What is hydramnios?

Excess of liquor amnios detected of any stage of pregnancy causing abnormality of pregnancy and labour.

SAQ 10 What are the etiologies of hydramnios?

Not known, more production and less absorption generally associated with:

- Monozygotic twins
- Diabetes mellitus
- Foetal malformation (an encephalic, spine bifida)
- Hydrops foetalis, chorioangioma. It may be acute, chronic or acute on chronic.

SAQ 11 What complications may arise out of hydramnios?

During pregnancy

- PET
- Premature labour
- Foetal malformation
- Malpresentation
- Non-engagement

During labour

- Inertia of uterus
- Early rupture of membrane and cord
- Retained placenta
- PPH

SAQ 12 What are the features of hydramnios?

Symptoms

- Breathlessness
- Enlarged abdomen
- Oedema.

Signs

- PET
- High BP
- Fundal height raised
- Fluid thrill present
- Foetal parts difficult to feel
- P/V bulging of membranes even in absence of pain

Investigations

- Radiology
- Fogged foetal shadow
- USG

15 Abnormal Umbilical Cord and Foetal Anomalies

SAQ 1 What is prolapse of umbilical cord?

When a loop of cord descent beside and below the maximum diameter of foetal presenting part is cord prolapse.

SAQ 2 What are the dangers of cord prolapse?

To mother

- Sepsis
- Haemorrhage

To foetus

- Asphyxia
- Spasm of cord
- Operative trauma to suboxygenated foetus

SAQ 3 How to treat cord prolapse?

Foetus is dead

Destructive operation of foetus with obstruction.

Foetus is alive

- Manual reposition of cord

  or
- Quick delivery if cervix in fully dilated
- Caesarean section.

SAQ 4 Mention some of the abnormalities of the umbilical cord.

- Abnormal length (above 30" or below 12")
- Abnormal insertion
- True knot
- Torsion of cord
- Neoplasm
- Inflammation
- Haematoma

SAQ 5 What is compound presentation?

When hand or foot presents or prolapses beside head.

SAQ 6 What are the causes of compound presentation?

- Twins
- Prematurity
- Contracted pelvis
- Hydramnios
- Foetal malformation
- Cephalic version

SAQ 7 Mention some important causes of large foetus.

- Postmaturity
- Diabetes
- Heredity

SAQ 8 What is anencephalus?

It is deficient development of brain and cranial vault. On diagnosis before 20 weeks, MTP is performed.

SAQ 9 What is hydrocephalus?

This congenital malformation occurs due to excess accumulation of CSF in ventricles of brain. Vaginal decompression or abdominal decompression is done to initiate labour.

SAQ 10 What is a Siamese twin?

The double monster or Siamese twins are conjoined twins delivered by elective caesarean section separated by operation afterwards if feasible (thoracopagus, dicephalus, etc.)

SAQ 11 What is oligohydramnios?

The scanty liquor amnii (less than 500 ml) causing abnormality in pregnancy. In placental insufficiency, pregnancy is to be terminated.

SAQ 12 What complications may arise out of oligohydramnios?

- Foetal abnormality
- Foetal pulmonary hypoplasia
- Breech presentation
- Uterine inertia

SAQ 13 Define: (i) Placenta succenturiate, (ii) Placenta membranous, (iii) Placenta circumvallata, (iv) Battledore placenta, (v) Velamentous insertion of placenta.

(i) **Placenta succenturiate:** Here one or more small accessory lobes of placenta away from main mass connected by membranes with umbilical vessels.
(ii) **Placenta membranous:** Thin and large placenta occupying large uterine wall.
(iii) **Placenta circumvallata:** Membranes attached away from placenta.
(iv) **Battledore placenta:** Cord is attached to the margins of placenta.
(v) **Velamentous insertion of cord:** It occurs from distance of placental margin.
(vi) Morbid adhesion up to deciduous is **placenta accreta**, up to muscle is **increta** and up to uterine wall is **percreta**.

16 Cephalopelvic Disproportion

SAQ 1 What is contracted pelvis?

The female bony pelvis, whose shape and size insufficient for vaginal delivery.

SAQ 2 What do you mean by disproportion?

Here baby is large for vaginal delivery. The reasons are:

(i) Large baby
(ii) Contracted pelvis
(iii) Combination of (i) and (ii).

SAQ 3 What are the different types of pelvis?

- Gynaecoid
- Android
- Anthropoid
- Platypelloid

SAQ 4 How to diagnose CPD?

- History (rickets, or pelvic disease)
- Obstetrical history
- General survey (height, gait, etc.)
- Abdominal exam(pendulous belly, non-engaged head, malpresentation; non-engaged head on standing)
- Vaginal examination to assess pelvis; Muller Kerr method
- X-ray for pelvimetry, sonographic pelvimetry

LAQ 5 What is Muller Kerr's method?

Patient position lithotomy, right thumb is placed in front of symphysis pubis. Left hand presses down head towards pelvis. The two fingers of right hand measures descent of head and the right thumb estimates overlapping of head on symphysis pubis. If head can enter pelvis, there is no CPD if head cannot pushed into pelvis then there is CPD.

SAQ 6 How to manage CPD?

(i) Premature induction of labour
(ii) Trial labour or
(iii) Caesarean section. All in hospitals under care of specialist.

SAQ 7 When not to go for trial labour in CPD?

(i) Elderly primi
(ii) Associated disease like kidney, hypertension, heart ailment
(iii) Malpresentation
(iv) Postmaturity

SAQ 8 What are the causes of floating head at term in primigravida?

- CPD
- Placenta previa
- Full bladder and rectum
- Ill-formed lower uterine segment
- Pelvic tumour
- Lower uterine caesarean segment
- Deflexed vertex, multiple pregnancy
- Hydramnios
- Pre- and postmaturity, hydrocephalus
- Large foetus

Abnormal Uterine Contraction

17

SAQ 1 What is prolonged labour?

Inefficient uterine action or prolong labour, dysfunction of labour called uterine inertia when dysfunction occurs from beginning, it is primary uterine inertia or if contraction is normal starting with and gradually ensuing inertia, it is called secondary uterine inertia.

SAQ 2 What are different types of uterine inertia?

(A) Hypotonic inertia	(B) Hypertonic uterine dysfunction	(C) Constriction ring	(D) Cervical dystocia
Commonest, infrequent feeble contraction, foetal distress appears late.	Uterine hypertonicity and inco-ordination, more distressing pain on back, ketosis may develop; membranes ruptures early and so does foetal distress.	Localized annular ring spasm, generally around neck of foetus. Foetal distress common. Forceps fails.	Cervical non-dilatation. There may be edematous anterior cervical lip or fibrous external os.

SAQ 3 What are the causes of abnormal uterine action?

- Elderly primi
- Short stocky woman
- Full bladder and rectum
- Multiparity
- Twins
- Hydramnios
- Fibroid
- Nervousness
- Injudicious use of anaesthetics
- NSAID
- Oxytocics

SAQ 4 What are the different types of uterine overactivity encountered in practice?

Uterine overactivity may be in the form of:

Retraction ring	Precipitate labour
Excessive retraction of upper segment and lower segment becomes thin, a ring appears at junction called Bandl's ring.	It is unusual quick labour due to uterine overactivity within three hours, may be due to overactivity, oxytocics with foetus in favourable position, lack of resistance in cervix.

SAQ 5 What are the causes of premature rupture of membranes?

- Friable membrane
- Idiopathic
- Chorioamnionitis
- CPD
- Malpresentation
- Twins
- Hydramnios
- Cervical incompetence
- Deliberately

LAQ 6 What are the favourable and unfavourable effects of early rupture of membrane?

Favourable	Unfavourable
It has been claimed to mature foetal lungs.	Dry labour, continuous leakage of amnii, prolong labour, prolapse of cord, infection, amniotic embolism.

SAQ 7 How to diagnose premature rupture?

- Characteristic smelling liquor leaking may be with meconium
- Alkaline pH
- Cytologically shows foetal cutaneous squamous cells
- Fat laden cells of foetus stains red with Nile blue
- Grasping of foetal scalp possible

SAQ 8 What are the causes of delay of second stage labour?

- Occipitoposterior, face, brow, breech, shoulder like malpresentations
- Inertia of uterus
- Constriction ring
- Twins
- Contracted pelvis
- Obstruction in vagina
- Ovarian tumour
- Improper anaesthesia
- Fibroid
- Full bladder and rectum

SAQ 9 What is elderly primi?

Woman going for pregnancy above 35 years of age.

SAQ 10 What is obstructed labour?

It is mechanical obstruction in the process of foetus delivery through normal passage may be due to constriction ring, bony passage defect (osteomalacia, android pelvis) soft tissue defect (fibroid, impacted ovarian cyst); large baby, defective presentation.

SAQ 11 Define grandmultipara.

Woman given birth to more than five viable babies.

SAQ 12 What is the obstetrical treatment of obstructed labour?

If diagnosed early, elective or emergency caesarean section or destructive operation depending upon cause.

18 Maternal Injuries in Labour

SAQ 1 Define vulval haematoma.

These are haemorrhage from paravaginal veins usually unilateral causing vulval swelling.

LAQ 2 What are causes of rupture of uterus?

Rupture of uterus means giving away of gravid uterus, may be complete up to peritoneal coat or incomplete. Etiologically, it may be classified as:

Spontaneous

- Caesarean section scar
- Hysterotomy scar
- Accidental haemorrhage
- Obstructed labour
- Misuse of oxytocic

Traumatic

- Accident
- External version
- Craniotomy
- Decapitation
- Forceps delivery
- Manual removal of placenta

SAQ 3 How to diagnose rupture uterus?

Symptoms

Pain, vaginal haemorrhage, history of oxytocic use.

Signs

Shock, tenderness, abdominal distension,vaginal haemorrhage

LAQ 4 How to manage post-caesarean section pregnancy?

Since the indications of caesarean section is always caesarean has been shifted to once caesarean always hospital delivery, and twice caesarean always caesarean. These patients require close observation during pregnancy and trial, vaginal delivery should be done in hospital set up (note pulse, BP; tender scar). Following vaginal delivery of baby and placenta, integrity of the lower uterine scar is noted, sterilization is generally advisable after third caesarean section.

SAQ 5 What are the different types of injuries seen after delivery?

Following types of maternal birth passage injury may occur in labour.

- Perineal tear
- Vaginal tear
- Vulval haematoma
- Cervical tear
- Rupture of uterus

19 Puerperium

SAQ 1 What is puerperium?

It is the six weeks period also called fourth trimester after delivery when maternal system return to pregravid state.

SAQ 2 Describe in brief the puerperium.

Pulse rate and temperature return to normal, hydraemia disappears, leukocytosis comes to normal, diuresis occurs, dilated ureter and renal pelvis come to normal. Endocrine glands regress. Involution of uterus and genital organ occurs; lochia dischage starts, vagina takes long time to involute. Ovulation starts after 11 weeks in non-lactators and 17 weeks in lactators. Menstruation starts in 7–9 weeks in non-lactators and by 36 weeks in lactators. Breast enlarges, hypertrophy and secretes colostrum, milk secretion starts from 3rd day of delivery.

LAQ 3 What is lochia?

It is physiological uterine discharge in postpartum period containing blood and necrotic deciduas lasting for 3–4 weeks of puerperium. For first 3–4 days, its colour is red called lochia rubra then fades yellow for one week called lochia serosa and ultimately whitish turbid called lochia alba persist for one week up to 4th week.

It is alkaline with peculiar smell, consisting of RBC, WBC, fibrin, decidual debris, peptone, vaginal epithelium, cholestrin crystals, may contain anaerobic *Strepto* and *Staphylo* which is normal in absence of clinical signs of sepsis.

SAQ 4 What is puerperal pyrexia?

Temperature above 100.4° F or more within 14 days of confinement, may be due to sepsis, UTI breast infection, bronchitis, pneumonia; PT, and other causes of fever, leg vein thrombosis.

LAQ 5 How to manage normal puerperium?

The management aims to provide mother's normal health, encourage breastfeeding and contraceptive, as follows with:

- Rest
- Adequate diet and calories
- Drugs (methergin, laxative, haematinics)
- Care of breast
- Care of perineum
- Control of infection by restricting visitors
- Posture and breathing exercises
- Rooming in
- Breastfeeding encouragement

SAQ 6 When and how to suppress lactation?

Baby is stillborne or there is other contraindications of breastfeeding. Done by wearing tight brassiere; ethynyl oestradiol (linoral) or oestrogen-androgen combination (mixogen) or testosterone oenanthate and oestradiol valerate (primodian depot 3 ml) or bromocriptine 2.5 mg BD × 2 weeks.

SAQ 7 What is puerperal sepsis?

It is the infection of genital tract either after child birth or abortion.

SAQ 8 Who was Semmelweis?

I.P. Semmelweis of Vienna first identified puerperal sepsis due to wound infection.

SAQ 9 What is subinvolution?

When involution process is deficient.

SAQ 10 What are the causes of subinvolution?

- Multiparity
- Overdistension as in twins or hydramnios
- APH

- Fibroid uterus
- Non-suckling baby
- Retention of placental bits
- Sepsis
- Retroverted uterus
- Lochiometra.

SAQ 11 What are the clinical features of subinvolution?

Symptoms

- Prolong discharge P/V
- After pain
- Fever

Signs

- Anaemia
- Patulous cervix.
- Large uterus may be with foeted discharge Uterus may be retroverted

Effects

- Ill health
- Prolapse
- Backache
- Retroversion
- Menorrhagia
- Dysmenorrhoea
- Leukorrhoea

SAQ 12 What is phlegmasia alba dolens?

It is iliofemoral thrombosis after extrapelvic spread of infection from pelvic thrombophlebitis producing indurated, painful, swollen white leg treated with:

- Rest
- Pain killer
- Antibiotics
- Anticoagulant heparin IV or dindevan orally
- Physiotherapy to start after relief of pain

SAQ 13 Mention some breast complications during puerperium.

- Mastitis
- Engorged breast on 3–4 days
- Cracked nipple
- Retracted nipple
- No lactation

SAQ 14 What are the clinical features of acute mastitis?

Here infection of glandular system of breast occurs derived from nasopharynx or cracked nipples, presents with:

Symptoms

High fever, rigor, malaise, unilateral breast pain.

Signs

Toxic; hard, knotty, red tender area on breast, draining axillary nodes are hard tender may prominent spenceris tail.

SAQ 15 What are the causes of failing lactation?

- Feeble premature baby
- Absent breastfeeding
- Ill health of mother with developmental defect of breast and nipple
- Apprehension.

SAQ 16 Mention some psychiatric diseases of pregnancy.

During pregnancy

- Anxiety neurosis
- Hysteria
- Psychosis
- Korsakoff psychosis

During labour

- Psychosis

20 Operations in Obstetrics

SAQ 1 What are the indications of P/V examination in obstetrics?

During pregnancy

- To confirm diagnosis and to detect fibroid cyst, cervical incompetence.
- Last two weeks to see CPD, abnormal presentation.

During labour

Onset of normal or abnormal labour and before obstetric operation.

During puerperium

At the end of 6th week.

> No P/V examination should be done in case of APH in outdoor.

LAQ 2 What are the different methods of induction of labour adopted before and after 12 weeks of pregnancy?

Up to 12 weeks

- D and C
- Vacuum aspiration

13–28 weeks

- Intra-amniotic hypertonic saline or urea
- Extra-amniotic ethacrydine lactate
- Syntocinon IV
- Prostaglandin
- Hysterotomy (abdominal or vaginal)

LAQ 3 What are the indications for induction of labour?

Deliberate induction of labour after 28 weeks for terminating pregnancy as urgency for mother and foetus.

INDICATIONS

Obstetrics

- PET
- APH
- Hydramnios
- Foetal malformation
- Post-dated or post-mature
- Growth retarded
- IUFD
- Rh incompatibility
- CPD
- Unstable lie

Maternal

- Hypertension
- Diabetes mellitus
- Chronic renal disease

LAQ 4 What are the different methods of induction of labour?

Medical

- Oil bath enema
- Syntocinon drip
- Prostaglandins
- Laminaria tent

Surgical

- Low rupture of membranes
- High rupture of membranes
- Stripping of membranes
- Combination of low rupture with syntocinon

SAQ 5 What are the risks of rupture of membranes?

- Cord prolapse
- Drainage of liquor
- Infection
- Injury to cervix

SAQ 6 What are the indications of episiotomy?

It is deliberate incision made on perineum to enlarge vaginal introitus in 2nd stage of labour to facilitate vaginal delivery indicated in:

- Primigravida with rigid perineum
- Persistent occipitoposterior
- Face

- Breech with aftercoming head
- Forceps delivery in primigravida. To cut short second stage of labour
- Perineal scar

Aimed to cut short second stage labour, foetal asphyxia, prevent genital prolapse and prevent perineum injury.

SAQ 7 What structures are cut inside outwards in episiotomy?

Posterior vaginal wall → deep and superficial perineal pouches with muscles (deep and superficial perineal muscle → transverse perineal muscle, levator ani) → superficial perineal fascia → skin.

SAQ 8 What is version?

It is the manipulation to alter foetal lie.

External

- Indicated for breech or shoulder into vertex or shoulder into breech.

Internal

(Always podalic)

- Shoulder presentation.
- Vertex with cord prolapse.

SAQ 9 What is vantouse?

Ventouse or vacuum extractor is device introduced by Malmstorm for extraction of head by suction traction as an alternative to forceps. Indicated in uterine inertia, or alternative to low forceps. Contraindicated for premature foetus and acute foetal distress.

LAQ 10 What is Bishop's score?

It is score to see cervical dilatation.

	Score '0'	Score '1'	Score '2'	Score '3'	Total
Dilatation	Closed	1–2 cm	3–4 cm	5 or more	0–3
Effacement	30%	40–50%	60–70%	80%	0–3
Station of head	– 3	– 2	– 1	+1 +2	0–3
Consistency	Firm	Medium	Soft	—	0–2
Position	Posterior	Mid	Anterior	—	0–2

For ARM, if score is more than 9, condition is favourable for induction, if less than 5, it is unfavourable.

SAQ 11 What are the indications of craniotomy?

This destructive operation on foetal head with perforation and extraction indicated for:

- CPD
- Foetal head malformation
- Impacted occipitoposterior

SAQ 12 What is decapitation?

In this destructive operation of dead foetus, neck is severed for vaginal delivery indicated in dead impacted shoulder presentation or locked twins for delivery of dead baby.

SAQ 13 What is evisceration?

In this destructive operation, foetal abdomen and thorax are opened by embryotomy, indicated for foetal ascitis, monster, impacted shoulder in dead foetus.

SAQ 14 What is cleidotomy?

Operation to divide one or both clavicles to deliver shoulder with narrow maternal pelvis.

SAQ 15 What are the indications of caesarean section?

It is the abdominal delivery of baby by laparotomy after 28 weeks when vaginal delivery is dangerous for mother and/or foetus.

- (A) **Uterine defect**
  - Inertia
  - Constriction ring
- (B) **Birth passage defect**
  - **Bony**
    - Rickets
    - Contraction
  - **Soft tissue**
    - Previous caesarean section
    - Fibroid
    - Cancer
    - Ovarian cyst
    - Vaginal atresia
- (C)
  - Big baby
  - Postmaturity
  - Foetal distress
- (D) **Others**
  - APH
  - Mother with disease

SAQ 16 What are the different types of caesarean section?

According to:

Operation type

- Lower uterine
- Classical upper uterine
- Caesarean hysterectomy

Operation time

- Emergency
- Elective

SAQ 17 What are the different indications of postpartum sterilization?

Postportum sterilization is done after caesarean section, hysterectomy (abdominal) or early puerperium indicated for following conditions.

Obstetric ground

- Repeat caesarean
- Osteomalacia repeat PET

Medical ground

- Heart disease
- Hypertension
- PT
- Diabetes of mother

Socioeconomic

- Population control

SAQ 18 What are the different types of obstetric forceps?

Obstetric forceps are designed for vaginal extraction of the foetus presenting by vertex or for after coming head in breech. They are commonly of following types:

- Das's long curved forceps
- Wrigley's short forceps
- Kielland's forceps

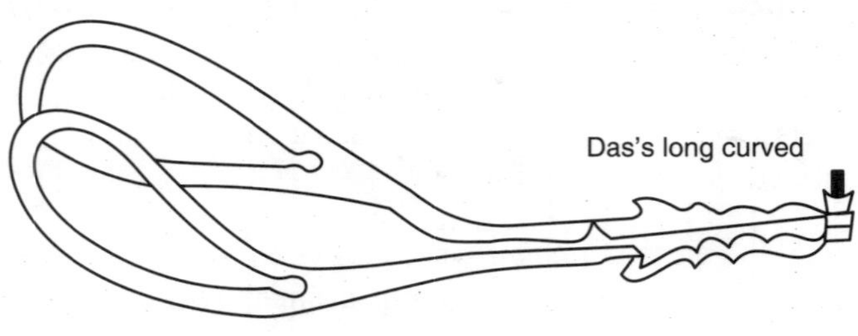

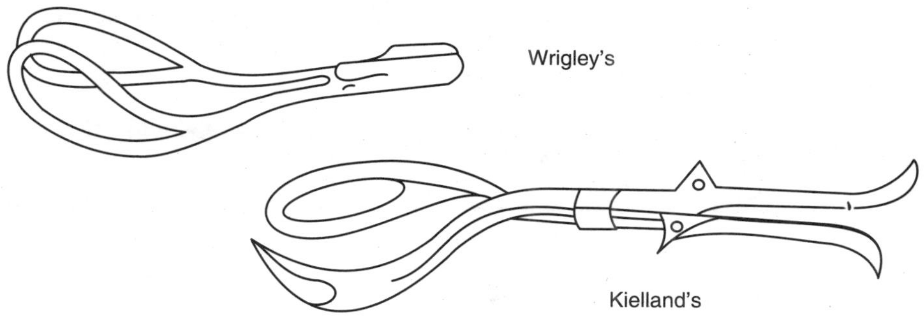

SAQ 19 What is trial forceps?

Trial forceps are applied on borderline outlet contraction with an idea for safe vaginal delivery.

SAQ 20 What criteria should be fulfilled before forceps operation?

- Cervix fully dilated
- Membrane must be ruptured
- Presentation should be vertex or after coming head if breech
- Sagittal suture should be in anteroposterior diameter
- Uterine contraction should be sufficient
- Baby should be alive

SAQ 21 How the forceps helps delivery?

It helps by:

- Traction
- Rotation
- Slight compression of head
- Stimulating uterine contraction.

SAQ 22 What are contraindications of forceps delivery?

- Undilated os
- CPD
- Uterine inertia
- Floating head
- Brow malpresentation

21 Drugs Acting on Uterus

SAQ 1 What is oxytocics/ecbolics/abortifacient?

The drugs which increase uterine motility at terms are called oxytocics, viz.:

1. Posterior pituitary extract – oxytocin.
2. Ergot alkaloids – Ergometrine or methylergometrine.
3. Prostaglandins – PGE_2, $PGF_{2\alpha}$; 5-methyl $PGF_{2\alpha}$; misoprostol.
4. Miscellaneous – quinine; ethacridine.

SAQ 2 What are the indications of oxytocins?

(i) In early pregnancy. Inevitable, incomplete, missed abortion, or hydatidiform mole.
(ii) In late pregnancy to induce labour.
(iii) During labour to accelerate the process and to prevent PPH and caesarean section.
(iv) Intranasal spray for milk ejection.
(v) Oxytocin challenge test to see uteroplacental adequacy.

SAQ 3 What are the dangers of oxytocins?

The dangers of oxytocins are:

- Rupture of uterus
- Foetal hypoxia or death
- Rupture uterus
- Shock

SAQ 4 What is to tocolytics?

These drugs decrease uterine motility used for delaying labour, threatened abortion, dysmenorrhoea, viz.:

(i) Adrenergic agonist (ritodrine, salbutamol)
(ii) Magnesium sulfate
(iii) Calcium channel blocker
(iv) PG-synthesis inhibitor
(v) Ethyl alcohol
(vi) Progesterone
(vii) Miscellaneous—anticholinergic, diazoxide, nitrites, general anaesthetics.

Section 2
Neonate Care

Care of the Newborn 22

SAQ 1 What immediate care should be taken after delivery?

(i) Immediate head down to drain liquor amnii and to clean mouth and nasopharynx
(ii) To see congenital defect
(iii) Baby bath
(iv) Cord dressing with (ZnO, boric acid, starch or tripledy)
(v) Clothing
(vi) Weighing
(vii) Feeding (encourage breastfeeding)

LAQ 2 What are the contraindications of breastfeeding?

Contraindications of breastfeeding are:

- Mastitis
- TB of mother
- Acute infection of mother
- Puerperal sepsis
- Epilepsy of mother on drugs
- Psychologically disturbed mother
- Ill baby
- Hare lip of baby
- Cleft palate of baby
- Premature baby

SAQ 3 Mention the conditions where breastfeeding can fail.

Breastfeeding may fail in:

(i) Retracted or sored or cracked nipple
(ii) Toxemic mother and caesarean baby
(iii) Elderly mother
(iv) Weak baby
(v) Undernourished mother
(vi) Mother's mental status

SAQ 4 What do you mean by demand and time schedule of breastfeeding?

Breastfeeding is given when baby is hungry (demand schedule). When given on specific time (time schedule).

SAQ 5 What is burping?

Burping or breaking up of wind is to be done after each breastfeeding by holding upright the baby on lap or shoulder and patting the baby at the back.

SAQ 6 How will you know breastfeeding is insufficient?

(i) No weight gain of baby
(ii) Constant crying between feeds and at night
(iii) Constipation.

SAQ 7 What is weaning?

Gradual change over from breastfeeding to solid food or cow's milk, the procedure is called weaning.

SAQ 8 What are the indications of artificial feeding?

(i) Ill mothers without sufficient milk.
(ii) Weak baby to suck.
(iii) Dried up mother's milk.

SAQ 9 How to humanize the cow's milk?

Cow's milk is diluted with equal amount of water, fat is removed and added in smaller amount or in unsaturated form. Carbohydrate is added to sweeten it to increase caloric value.

SAQ 10 What are the indications of exchange transfusion?

(i) Bilirubin more than 3 gm and cord blood Hb 14.8 gm or direct Coombs' test positive.
(ii) Premature baby with Hb less than 14.8 gm + direct Coombs' positive and bilirubin 3 gm.
(iii) History of hydrops foetalis.
(iv) Bilirubin rising 0.5 mg% per hour in first 24 hours.

> Exchanged blood should be Rh negative of same ABO group.

LAQ 11 What is Apgar score?

This is a method generally adopted to determine neonatal asphyxia at birth at one minute and five minutes after complete birth. Score 0,1,2 are given to the following signs.

Signs	0	1	2
Effect for respiration	Absent	Slow	Good; crying
Heart rate	Absent	Below 100	Over 100
Muscle tone	Nil	Some flexion	Active
Reflex on touching catheter to nose	Nil	Grimace	Cough and sneezing
Colour	White	Pink body extremities blue	Completely pink

Score 0–3 (severe depression; asphyxia pallida). 4–6 (mild depression, asphyxia livida).

LAQ 12 What are the causes of neonatal jaundice?

(I) Increased haemolysis
- ABO; Rh immunization
- Spherocytosis
- Glucose 6-PO_4 dehydrogenase deficiency
- Septicaemia
- Hb pathy
- Excess vitamin K
- Sulfonamide drug

(II) Liver cell defect
- Gilbert's disease.

(III) Defective conjugation
- Physiological
- Crigler-Najjar syndrome.

(IV) Failure to excrete conjugated bilirubin
- Hepatitis
- Portal pyemia
- Galactosaemia
- Congenital atresia of bile duct

(V) Miscellaneous
- Hypothyroid
- Down syndrome
- Intestinal obstruction

SAQ 13 What are the causes of hydrops foetalis?

The causes of oedematous stillborne baby (hydrops foetalis) are:
- Severe anaemia
- Cardiac failure due to congenital heart disease

- Polycystic kidney
- Diabetes
- Umbilical vein thrombosis
- Chorioangioma of placenta

SAQ 14 Mention some marketed canned milk.

Lactogen, Amul, Amul spray, Glaxo, Ostermilk, Madhuspray (full cream); Raptakos infant food (humanised milk with-unsaturated fatty acids); Lactodex (skimmed milk) Amul whole milk, Nespray (whole milk); Balamul, Cerelac, Lactogen milk cereals (Cereal with milk).

LAQ 15 Mention the immunization schedule.

At birth – BCG + OPV (first dose)
At 6–10–14 weeks – DPT + OPV.
At 12 months – measles
At 15–18 months – DPT + OPV (booster).
At 5 years (school entry) DT; OPV booster typhoid (TAB 2 doses)
At 10 years – tetanus toxoid + typhoid (optional).
For pregnant women – tetanus toxoid 16–24 weeks or 24–36 weeks.

Section 3
Gynaecology

- Some Diagnostic Methods in Gynaecology
- Puberty and Menopause
- Disorders of Menstruation
- Retroversion of Uterus, Genital Prolapse and Hypertrophy of Cervix
- Infertility; Vaginismus; Dyspareunia, Frigidity
- Fertility Control
- Diagnosis of Sex; Intersex, Virilism, Hirsutism
- Complete Perineal Tear, Uterine Inversion; RVF
- Urinary Incontinence and Genitourinary Fistula
- Pelvic Inflammatory Diseases
- Uterine Fibroid and Endometriosis
- Malignancies of Genital Tract
- Ovarian Tumours/Radiotherapy/ Chemotherapy
- Backache, Pruritus Vulvae; Leukorrhoea
- Paediatric and Geriatric Gynaecology
- Oestrogen and Progesterone Hormone Therapy
- Operations in Gynaecology

Some Diagnostic Methods in Gynaecology

23

LAQ 1 Mention the important cytological diagnostic methods in gynaecology.

Following are important cytological diagnostic methods in gynaecology:

For genital cancer	Cytohormonal diagnosis	Sex determination	Fluid aspiration of cyst; ascitis, etc.
(i) Vaginal pool aspiration. (ii) Cervical scrapping by Ayre's spatula. (iii) Vacuum curatte aspira--tion from cervix or endometrial canal.	Scrapped from upper lateral vaginal wall to see hormonal influence.	Scrapped from buccal mucosa, leucocyte for extrachromatin mass.	Aspirated fluid stained by PAP stain for cancer cells.

SAQ 2 What is PAP stain?

It consists of three dyes.

(1) Haematoxylin for staining nucleus.
(2) Orange G.
(3) Mixture of Bismark brown; eosin yellow and light green. The cytoplasm of mature cells, take orange G and eosin. The less mature cells stain by light green.

SAQ 3 What is colposcopy?

It is optical diagnostic instrument magnifies vaginal cervix 10–40 times Colpomicroscope magnifies the same up to 100–300 times.

SAQ 4 What are the indications of colposcope?

It helps localization of suspicious cancer so that biopsy can be taken indicated for:

(i) Follow up of benign lesion, (ii) Recurrence of lesion of cervix after radiotherapy.

SAQ 5 What are the disadvantages of colposcope?

- Preclinical and intracervical cancer can be missed
- False postive dysplasia
- Requires sophisticated instrument and trained personnel
- Time consuming

SAQ 6 Who introduced colposcope?

Hinselmann of Hamburg.

SAQ 7 What is gynaecography?

The pelvic viscera are demonstrated by producing pneumoperitoneum by X-rays.

LAQ 8 How the pneumoperitoneum is produced?

It is done either by transabdominal or transuterine route if fallopian tube are patent. For transabdominal route, an area one inch below and left of umbilicus is infiltrated with 1% lignocaine and 18 gauze LP needles with stylet or Verres needle is introduced into peritoneal cavity at 45° and connected to source of gas (nitrous oxide, O_2 or CO_2 about 1–1.5L or room air) with slightly head down.

After the X-ray is taken, patient goes to bed and sits for 2 hours and can be discharged home after 4 hours, if there is discomfort then foot end is raised.

SAQ 9 How the stained smear is graded after Papanicolaous classification?

Grade I: Normal negative smear
Grade II: Atypical cases as like infection and metaplasia
Grade III: Suspicious atypical smear
Grade IV: Positive smear with dysplasia
Grade V: Positive smear with large number of malignant cells.

LAQ 10 What are the indications and contraindications of gynaecography?

Indications

(i) Stein-Leventhal syndrome
(ii) Amenorrhoea (primary and secondary)
(iii) Mass in pelvis, myoma, double uterus

Contraindications

(i) PID
(ii) Pregnancy (transuterine pneumoperitoneum)
(iii) Cardiorespiratory disease
(iv) Large pelvic tumour

SAQ 11 Name some endoscopic instruments for gynaecology.

(i) Laparoscopy, (ii) culdoscopy, (iii) hysteroscopy.

SAQ 12 What is laparoscopy?

It is an endoscopic instrument for visualization of peritoneal cavity through anterior abdominal walls after producing pneumoperitoneum.

SAQ 13 Why pneumoperitoneum is produced before laparoscopy?

It pushes away the intestine from abdominal wall for better visualization of pelvic organs.

LAQ 14 What are the indications and contraindications of laparoscopy?

Indications

(i) Detecting tubal morphology, patency
(ii) Evaluating ovulation by corpus luteum
(iii) Pre- and post-tuboplasty.
(iv) To diagnoses, pelvic TB; and PID
(v) Sterilization

Contraindications

(i) Cardiorespiratory disease
(ii) Obesity
(iii) Previous abdominal surgery
(iv) Acute PID
(v) Hernia's (hiatus, diaphragmatic, inguinal umbilical)

LAQ 15 What is hysteroscopy? What are its indications and contraindications?

It is fibro-optic endoscopic instrument for visualization of endometrial surface and uterotubal opening.

Indicated for

Diagnostic

- Polyp
- Fibroid
- Adhesion
- Septum
- IUCD

Therapeutic

- Cautery
- Biopsy
- Removal of IUCD

Contraindicated for

- PID
- Pregnancy
- Endometrial Ca
- Uterine bleeding

LAQ 16 What are the indications and contraindications of culdoscopy?

It is done in knee-chest position only.

Indicated for

Diagnostic
- Infertile woman
- Amenorrhoea
- Intersex
- PID
- Virilism
- Hirsutism

Therapeutic

Female sterilization.

Contraindicated for
- Retroverted uterus
- Occluded pouch of Douglas
- PID
- Vaginitis and cervicitis
- Ruptured ectopic gestation
- Children and aged
- Cannot adopt knee chest position

SAQ 17 Mention some of the applications of USG in gynaecology.

It helps in detection of:

- Uterine anomalies, fibroid
- Ovarian cyst and ascitis
- Intraperitoneal metastasis
- In obstetric cases

24 Puberty and Menopause

SAQ 1 Define puberty.

Latin word *pubertas* means adulthood is the period when sexual maturity occurs in girl. It starts at 8 years completes by 16 years.

SAQ 2 Define adolescence.

Latin word *adolescere* means to grow is the period between puberty and maturity. Here girl grows to adult woman with physical, sexual and psychosexual maturity.

SAQ 3 What is precocious puberty?

If a girl maturates and menstruates before 9th year, it is called precocious puberty.

SAQ 4 What is delayed puberty?

When a girl does not maturates and menstruates before 16 years of age, it is called delayed puberty.

SAQ 5 What is menstruation?

(Greek *men* = month) Menstruation is monthly vaginal bleeding coming periodically of about 28 days in menarche to menopause in normal woman except during pregnancy and lactation in oestrogen progesterone primed uterus.

The menstruation cycle starts from 1st day of cycle and continues till next phase of blood sheeding. It is devided into four phases: (i) post-menstrual phase, (ii) proliferative phase, (iii) secretory or pre-menstrual phase, (iv) menstrual phase.

SAQ 6 What is menarche?

It is the age of onset of first menstruation (10–16 years).

LAQ 7 Describe in brief the endocrine mechanism of menstruation.

Hormones from hypothalamus, anterior pituitary and ovary influence menstruation directly and thyroid and adrenal cortex hormone indirectly influence menstruation. The changes in uterine endometrium during menstrual cycle occur under influence of estrogen produced by theca interna and by interstitial gland cells. Progesterone is secreted by corpus luteum. Hormones of anterior pituitary hormones FSH (stimulates formation of follicles and secretion of oestrogen), LH (helps to convert ovarian follicle into corpus luteum which secretes progesterone), respectively. Ovulation is caused by LH surge occurs 30–36 hours after LH peak.

LAQ 8 Mention the cyclical changes in hormone level in menstrual cycle.

Rise in FSH during ovulation and menstruation up to 30 mIU/ml otherwise throughout the cycle it is 5–15 mIU/ml.

LH at ovulatory surge rises to 120 mIU/ml up to 24 h from 10 mIU/ml at follicular phase.

Plasma oestrogen, rises up to 500 pg/ml before ovulation from 100–200 pg/ml.

Plasma progesterone rising to 15 ng/ml during luteal phase from 1 ng/ml during follicular phase.

LAQ 9 Why there is menstrual bleeding?

(A) Due to withdrawal of hormones, the regressed functional layer of endometrium undergoes ischaemic necrosis due to vascular injury of coiled endometrial vessels. The bleeding occurs as:

- (i) Capillary bleeding
- (ii) Subepithelial haematoma under the necrosed endometrium
- (iii) Venous haemorrhage
- (iv) Diapedesis

(B) Stasis of circulation causing necrobiosis.

(C) Liberated prostaglandins producing vasospasm.

LAQ 10 Describe the clinical features of normal menstruation.

Menstruation is normal process, the discomforts of menstruation is called menstrual molimina.

- (i) Heavyness and discomfort in pelvis, lower abdomen.
- (ii) Pricking and fullness of breast.
- (iii) Constipation and urinary frequency.
- (iv) Depression; headache.
- (v) Rarely vicarious menstruation.

- (i) Fall in temperature, pulse rate and BP.
- (ii) Weight gain up to 1 kg
- (iii) Menstrual loss.

SAQ 11 What is the interval and duration of menstruation?

Average – 28 days, with a deviation of 2–3 days. However, with the possible deviation of 2–7 days, it may vary from 21 to 35 days.

SAQ 12 What is the amount of blood loss in menstruation?

5–60 ml on an average 35 ml; 2 fresh pads in a day and one at night (3 pads/day). Total 12–15 pads per menstruation.

LAQ 13 How to prepone or postpone menstruation?

Preponement and postponement are necessary due to some social reasons, can be done with hormone like:

(i) Progesterone – Norethisterone (Primolut – N) to be taken 1tab TDS from 20th day till the date of postponement.

(ii) Oestrogen progesterone contraceptive pills, taken BD started on 20th day till the date of postponement. Menstruation starts after 2–3 days. In order to prepone, the menstruation, therapy is started on 5th day to 14th day, with ethinyl oestradione 0.05 mg TDS or oestrogen – progesterone oral pill daily, menstrual flow starts after 2–3 days of stoppage of therapy.

SAQ 14 What is menopause?

It is the final cessation of menstruation.

LAQ 15 Describe the characteristics of menstrual loss.

The P/V bleeding of menstruation is dark reddish liquid (not clotted) mainly arterial, partly venous with disagreeable smell due to valvular sebaceous glands and decomposed blood. It is rich in calcium but deficient in prothrombin and fibrinogen factors. It contains RBC; WBC, cervical mucus, vaginal epithelium, macrophages, fragments of endometrium, mast cells, histiocytes, bacteria, cholesterol, PG, oestrogen. The clotted menstrual blood of endometrium is dissolved by fibrinolysin but clot may be passed if bleeding is excessive.

SAQ 16 What is climacteric?

It is the period when the woman gradually changes from reproductive life to senescence.

SAQ 17 What is the etiology of menopause?

Oestrogen deprivation due to ovarian failure.

SAQ 18 Mention the important physiological changes of menopause.

Genitals shows atrophy, ovary becomes fibrotic and smaller fallopian tube shrinks with decreased motility; uterus atrophies, vaginal smear shows atrophic changes with narrow introitus, supporting tissue becomes lax. Breast becomes flabby, pubic and axillary hairs are sparse, subcutaneous fat deposits on thigh, skin wrinkles, hyperlipidaemia and osteoporosis occurs. Emotional upset, gonadal failure.

LAQ 19 What are the clinical features of menopause?

Symptoms

- Either progressive scanty menstruation or menstruation at prolonged interval or sudden cessation. Prior cycles are anovular
- Weight gain
- Joint pain
- Increase sexual desire followed by fall
- Uterus body small and hard and ovaries are not palpable

Signs

- Fat deposited in hip, buttock, breast with weight gain.
- Vagina narrow, tenting, thin.
- Vulva atrophied with scanty hair.
- Atrophy of vaginal portion of cervix.

SAQ 20 What are the favourable and non-favourable points of hormone replacement therapy for menopause with oestrogen-progesterone contraceptive pills?

Favourable

Feels better; atrophic changes of external genitalia are less; conception control, prevent atherosclerosis, osteoporosis and vasomotor symptoms.

Non-favourable

Adverse effect on lipid profile and carbohydrate intolerance, coagulation producing thromboembolism, hypertension. Carcinogenic effect (breast, genitals, endometrium).

LAQ 21 What is menopausal syndrome?

It is group of symptoms experienced by few women during climacteric.
Symptoms are:

(i) Cessation of menstruation
(ii) Hot flushes in face and neck followed by sweating

(iii) Irritability
(iv) Sleepiness
(v) Giddiness
(vi) Depression
(vii) Fatigue
(viii) Pins and needles in palm
(ix) Constipation
(x) Joint pains

SAQ 22 How to diagnose menopausal syndrome?

(i) History
(ii) Clinical feature
(iii) Atrophic vaginal smear
(iv) Elevated urinary gonadotrophin

It has to be differentiated from pseudocyesis or pregnancy

25 Disorders of Menstruation

SAQ 1 What is amenorrhoea?

Where there is failure of menstruation.

LAQ 2 What are the different types of amenorrhoea?

It may be classified as following.

Classification-I

- **Physiological**
  1. Before puberty or after menopause.
  2. Pregnancy.
  3. At lactation.
- **Pathological**
  1. Disorder of menstrual flow.
  2. Environmental stress.
  3. Diseases of ovary, pituitary CNS; hypothalamus.

Classification-II

- **Primary**

  (No menarche up to 18 years.)
  1. Congenital obstruction.
  2. Rokitansky-Kuster-Hauser syndrome
  3. Defective uterine development
  4. Faulty gonadal development
     - Turner's syndrome
     - Intersex
  5. Adrenogenital syndrome.
  6. Juvenile diabetes mellitus.
  7. Pituitary dwarfism.
  8. Fröhlich's syndrome.
  9. Meningitis, fracture skull epilepsy.
  10. Undernutrition; malabsorption.
  11. Drugs (viz. anabolic steroid, androgens).
- **Secondary**

  Stoppage of menarche after few normal cycle.
  1. Pregnancy.
  2. Stenosis of outflow
  3. Hysterectomy.
  4. Tuberculosis of uterus
  5. Asherman's syndrome.
  6. Oophorectomy.
  7. Persistant corpus luteal cysts.
  8. Stein-Leventhal syndrome.
  9. Adrenogenital syndrome.
  10. Cushing's syndrome.
  11. Diabetes.
  12. Acromegaly.
  13. Simmonds' disease.

14. Psychogenic (pseudocyesis, anorexia, psycosis)
15. Infection.
16. Malnutrition.
17. Drugs (OCP: Androgen; Pb poisoning, alcohol and addiction.

SAQ 3 What is cryptomenorrhoea?

The concealed menstruation is called cryptomenorrhoea.

SAQ 4 What are the different causes of cryptomenorrhoea?

It may be classified as follows:

Congenital

(i) Imperforate hymen.
(ii) Atrasia of vagina.
(iii) Transverse vaginal septum.

Acquired

(i) Stenosis of cervix.

LAQ 5 What are the clinical features of cryptomenorrhoea?

Symptoms

- Urinary retention
- Constipation.
- Lower abdomen pain in teen-aged girl few days per month.
- Amenorrhoea.
- Swelling of lower abdomen.

Signs

- Well-developed secondary sex characters.
- P/A: Hypogastric swelling haematocolpos; Haematometra or haematosalpnix can be felt.
- P/V: Bulge bluish imperforate hymen seen.
- P/R: Tense vagina can be felt.

SAQ 6 What is Rokitansky-Kuster-Hauser syndrome?

This syndrome is characterised by:

(i) 46 XX karyotyping
(ii) Normal ovaries
(iii) Absent vagina and uterus is rudimentary
(iv) Kidney abnormal

SAQ 7 What are the features of Turner's syndrome?

Karyotyping 45 XO; short statured, cubitis vulgus, webbing of neck, congenital heart disease, (coarctation of aorta), infantile genital tracts, ovarian aplasia.

SAQ 8 What is Asherman's syndrome?

Cervical stenosis as a result of postpartum or postabortal intrauterine adhesion (synechial).

SAQ 9 What is Stein-Leventhal syndrome or polycystic ovarian disease?

This syndrome is characterised by the following in women: (i) bilateral large white polycystic ovaries, (ii) secondary amenorrhoea, (iii) infertility.

SAQ 10 What is Simmonds' disease?

This panhypopituitarism occurs as a result of necrosis or infarction of anterior pituitary gland characterised by cachexia, debility, amenorrhoea, hypotension, hypoglycaemia, low BMR; low 17 ketosteroid in urine; regression of genital organs.

Partial necrosis of anterior pituitary due to obstetric shock and PPH is called Sheehan's disease.

SAQ 11 What is hypomenorrhoea?

Hypomenorrhoea is scanty menstruation in duration and amount mostly nonpathological, requires only assurance or treatment like amenorrhoea.

SAQ 12 What is oligomenorrhoea?

If infrequent menstruation occurs at interval longer than 35 days, it is called oligomenorrhoea. Investigated like amenorrhoea.

LAQ 13 How to investigate a case of amenorrhoea?

(i) **History taking:** Age, pregnancy, cryptomenorrhoea, family history, menstrual history, history of TB, obstetric history of (PPH or shock) epilepsy, drug (OCP; anabolic steroids)

(ii) **General examination:** Nutrition secondary sex characters, pelvic exam: genitalia, pubic hair, imperforate hymen, adenexa exam, pregnancy ovarian tumour.

(iii) **Investigations:** Blood TC/DC/ESR/Hb% blood sugar (PP) urinalysis; D and C; and hysterogram, CXR (PA); T_3, T_4 and TSH, ophthalmoscopy for pituitary tumour, chromosome study, CT scan.

(iv) **Therapeutic hormone test:** (a) Progesterone challenge test: There will be withdraw bleeding if medroxyprogesterone acetate (Farlutal) 5 mg. BD × 5 days, i.e. intact hypothalamopituitary ovary uterus axis.(b) Oestrogen – progesterone challenge test: Withdrawn after giving for 20 days will lead to bleeding suggesting uterus is responsive . (c) Clomiphene challenge test: Clomiphene citrate – 100 mg daily × 7 days will rise FSH and LH suggesting intact pituitary. (d) LH/FSH-RH challenge test: There will be rise of plasma LH and FSH if IV. gonadotropines releasing hormones are given. (e) Hormone assay: Hormones FSH; prolactin, androgens, urinary 17 ketosteroid, plasma cortisol, etc. are assayed.

SAQ 14 Define dysmenorrhoea.

Dysmenorrhoea is painful menstruation, may interrupt educational, social life.

SAQ 15 What are the types of dysmenorrhoea?

Primary/intrinsic/functional/ spasmodic essential	Secondary/extrinsic/ organic/congestive
No pelvic lesion.	With pelvic lesion, viz. endometriosis, IUCD; PID, etc.

SAQ 16 What is membraneous dysmenorrhoea?

This variety of spasmodic dysmenorrhoea, generally runs in families where there is casting of big pieces of endometrium.

SAQ 17 What are the causes of pain in dysmenorrhoea?

A. For primary dysmenorrhoea: (i) obstruction, (ii) neurogenic, (iii) hypoplasia of uterus, (iv) nutritional, (v) psychogenic with low pain threshold, (vi) endocrine (ovular menstruation with progesterone), (vii) PG $F_2\alpha$.
B. For secondary dysmenorrhoea: (i) PID, (ii) fibroid, (iii) endometriosis.

SAQ 18 What is the prognosis of dysmenorrhoea?

Primary dysmenorrhoea generally cured after childbirth. Dysmenorrhoea developing after marriage persist till 30 years of age, secondary dysmenorrhoea appears late.

LAQ 19 Describe the clinical features of primary and secondary dysmenorrhoeas.

CLINICAL FEATURES

- **Primary dysmenorrhoea**
  - **Symptoms**: Young (18–24) starts after menarche, pain starts 2 hrs earlier of mens, last 24 hrs colicky (towards thigh) with no intermenstrual symptoms. There may be vomiting, fainting.
  - **Signs**: Poor health, anxious. No P/V or P/R or P/A finding.
- **Secondary dysmenorrhoea**
  - **Symptoms**: Elderly; painful mens after painless mens, starts 3–5 days before mens; on back, or lower abdomen, there may be white discharge, infertility, menorrhagia.
  - **Signs**: Anaemic PV/PR or PA shows pathology.

SAQ 20 How to treat primary dysmenorrhoea?

1. Sex education.
2. Medical treatment.
   - Rest.
   - Analgesic; antispasmodic.
   - Treatment of anaemia.
   - Hormones (oestrogen and progesterone to make cycle anovular from 5–25 days for six cycles, helpful for membranes dysmenorrhoea.)
   - Surgical: (a) D/C, (b) presacral neurectomy (Cotte's operation), (c) hysterectomy.

For secondary dysmenorrhoea treat the cause.

SAQ 21 What is mid-menstrual pain?

The pelvic pain occurring middle of menstruation regularly due to ovulation treated with analgesics or OCP (oestrogen-progesterone) to make the cycle anovular.

LAQ 22 What is premenstrual tension?

It is state that some women suffer form symptoms of irritability, lassitude, insomnia, headache, nausea, constipation, diarrhoea, oedema, pain in breast, epilepsy before childbirth 7–10 days before onset of menstruation.

Etiology is believed to be: (i) psychosomatic, (ii) salt and water retention due to oestrogen and progesterone, (iii) secondary hyperaldosteronism.

Treatment: (i) Salt and water restriction, (ii) diuretic, (iii) purgative, (iv) progesterone duphaston, or primolut N 5 mg, TDS or methyltestosterone 5 mg sublingual, TDS for sick days to improve tender breast symptoms, (v) Assurance, phenobarbitone or meprobamate or bromocriptine 2.5 mg TDS.

SAQ 23 What is epimenorrhoea?

Epimenorrhoea is frequent menstruation, heavy in amount at regular interval of 2–3 weeks. The etiologies are: (i) hyperactive anterior pituitary, (ii) malnutrition, (iii) asthenia, (iv) psychological, (v) PID, (vi) chocolate cyst of ovary.

SAQ 24 What is menorrhagia?

This is excessive menstruation in amount or duration or both.

SAQ 25 What is menotaxis?

Menotaxis is prolonged menstruation in duration.

SAQ 26 What is metrorrhagia?

It means intermenstrual irregular uterine bleeding.

SAQ 27 What is metrostaxis?

Metrostaxis is irregular haemorrhage before puberty or after menopause.

SAQ 28 What are the etiologies of menorrhagia?

These can be categorized as follows:

Causes in pelvis	Disorders of endocrine	General diseases
PID (tubercular endometritis, salpingo-oophoritis), fibroid, endometriosis, ovarian tumour, Ca endometrium; IUCD; malformation of uterus.	Hypo- and hyperthyroidism, DUB.	Hypertension, nephritis, CCF, anaemia, leukaemia, aspirin anticoagulants, worry, sexual excess.

SAQ 29 What is dysfunctional uterine haemorrhage (DUB)?

Any abnormal uterine haemorrhage (menorrhagia, polymenorrhoea, continuous bleeding) metrorrhagia) where no organic, systemic, haematological or pelvic cause is detected.

SAQ 30 What are the different types of haemorrhage of DUB?

It may be:

(I) Regular (ovular)

In the form of menorrhagia, polymenorrhoea. Curetting and suction of endometrium is normal.

(II) Irregular bleeding from irregular luteal phase

(III) Irregular/anovular

(i) Endometrial hyperplasia.
(ii) Proliferative endometrium.
(iii) Adenomatous hyperplasia.
(iv) Metropathia haemorrhagica (Schroeder's disease).

SAQ 31 What are the clinical features of DUB?

It occurs in reproductive age group, presents with:

Symptoms

Prolonged painless bleeding, menorrhagia Polymenorrhoea, symptoms of anaemia (palpitation, weakness).

Signs

Anaemia, uterus is normal by P/V or P/R. May be bulky in cystic ovary.

SAQ 32 How to investigate DUB?

The following should be investigated for DUB.

(i) Curettage from endometrium.
(ii) Haematological for Hb%; platelet count, BT; CT; TLC count for leukemia.
(iii) Vaginal and cervical smear to rule out carcinoma of oestrogen.
(iv) Hormonal assay and urinary 17 ketosteroid, PBI; T_3, T_4, TSH estimation.

SAQ 33 How to treat DUB?

The bleeding should be controlled and cyclical bleeding should be encouraged and this can be achieved by:

Medical therapy

(i) Rest, correction of anaemia; thyroxine for hypothyroidism.
(ii) Methergin, EACA, blood transfusion.
(iii) Hormone
- Oestrogen (rarely used).
- Progesterone (medical curettage).
- Oestrogen and progesterone.
- Androgen.

(iv) Clomiphene.
(v) Pregnancy.

Surgical therapy

(i) Dilatation and curettage.
(ii) Utriculoplasty or hysteroplasty.
(iii) Perimenopausal group with hysterectomy or radiotherapy.

LAQ 34 What are the causes of postmenopausal bleeding?

Any irregular bleeding per vagina after 6 months of menopause is postmenopausal bleeding, the etiologies are:

(i) Benign and malignant neoplasm of cervix.
(ii) Oestrogen therapy to treat menopause.
(iii) Ovarian neoplasm.
(iv) DUB.
(v) Injuries (decubitus ulcer; procidentia, pessary).
(vi) Infections (vagiitis; pyometra)
(vii) Blood dyscrasia.
(viii) Hypertension.
(ix) Haemorrhage from urinary bladder; rectum mistaken for vaginal bleeding.

26 Retroversion of Uterus, Genital Prolapse and Hypertrophy of Cervix

SAQ 1 What is retroversion of uterus?

When the uterus is retroflexed backwards along transverse axis through uterovaginal junction, it is called retroversion of uterus.

SAQ 2 What is the normal position of uterus?

Anteverted, anteflexed with external os directed down and back.

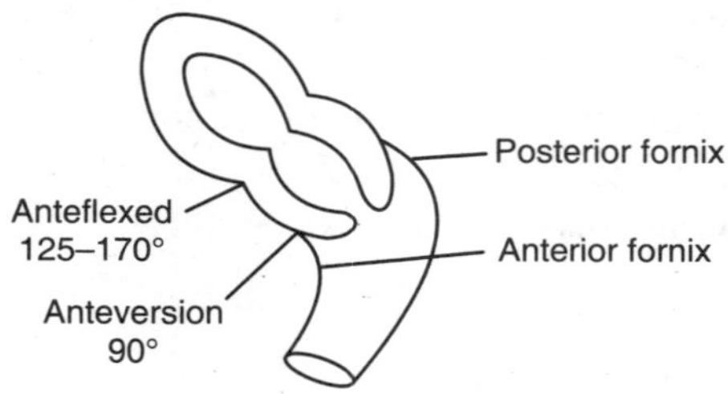

SAQ 3 What is retroflexion of uterus?

When the uterus body is bend on cervix, it is called retroflexion.

SAQ 4 What are the different types of retroversion?

According to degrees

1st° Fundus directed towards sacral promontory.
2nd° Fundus in hollow of sacrum.
3rd° Fundus lies below the level of internal os.

According to clinical types

1. Mobile retroversion.
2. Fixed retroversion.
3. Complicated retroversion with TO mass or prolapse.

SAQ 5 What are the causes of retroversion?

(i) Congenital

(ii) Acquired:

- (a) Puerperal
- (b) Prolapse of uterus
- (c) Pressure by tumour
- (d) Endometriosis
- (e) PID.

SAQ 6 What are the clinical features of prolapse?

Symptoms

- May be symptomless or backache
- Menstrual disorders
- Infertility
- Leukorrhoea
- Dyspareunia.

Signs

P/V shows:

- Cervix directed downward and forward.
- Body of uterus not palpable from anterior fornix.
- Adnexal disease P/R confirms P/V findings.

SAQ 7 How to treat retroversion of uterus?

Symptomless retroversion requires reassurance and no treatment otherwise it is treated by: (a) pessary or (b) surgery.

SAQ 8 What are the indications and contraindications of pessary?

Indications

(i) Mobile retroversion with pessary test positive as in puerperal or gravid uterus.

Contra-indications

(i) Fixed retroversion.

(ii) Perineal relaxation.

(iii) PID.

SAQ 9 What is genital prolapse?

When pelvic organs herniates through vagina, viz. (a) Cystocele: Prolapse of urinary bladder through anterior vaginal wall, (b) Rectocele: Prolapse of rectum with part of posterior vaginal wall, (c) Urethrocele: Prolapse of urethra with part of anterior vaginal wall, (d) Enterocele: Prolapse of pouch of Douglas with upper third of vaginal wall, (e) Uterine prolapse: Descending of uterus P/V may of vaginouterine type or uterovaginal type.

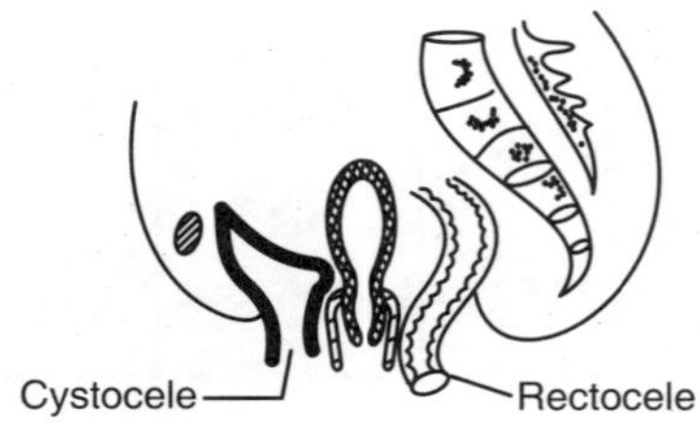

SAQ 10 What are the different degrees of uterine prolapse?

1st degree

Cervix descends from normal position.

2nd degree

Cervix goes out of vagina but uterus lies inside.

3rd degree

Uterus is out of vagina.

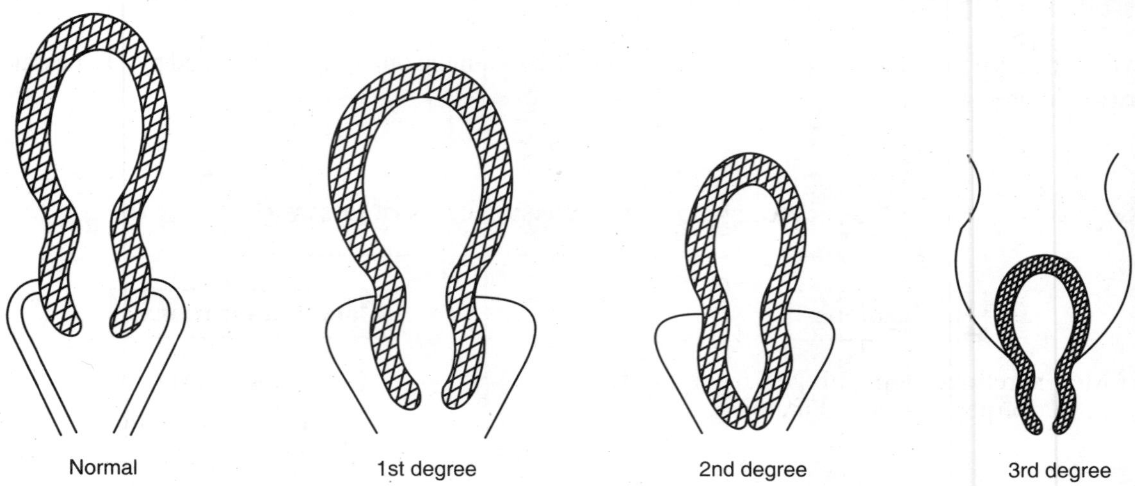

SAQ 11 What are the causes of prolapse?

Failure of pelvic organs support

- Congenital
- Acquired
  - Birth trauma.
  - Atrophy
  - Surgery

Raised abdominal pressure

- Cough, constipation, dysentery, weight lifting.
- Uterine fibroid or bulky uterus.

SAQ 12 What are the complications of uterine prolapse?

(i) Vaginal mucosa is thickened, dry, pigmented.
(ii) Decubitus ulcer
(iii) Infection.
(iv) Hypertrophic elongation of cervix.

SAQ 13 What are structures encountered in procidentia before backwards?

- Anterior vaginal wall
- Urinary bladder
- Uterovesicle pouch
- Uterus
- Pouch of Douglas
- Posterior vaginal wall.

SAQ 14 Describe the clinical features of prolapse.

Symptoms

- Something coming down P/V
- Backache
- White discharge
- Urinary frequency with difficulties in emptying
- Stress incontinence
- Constipation

Signs

Child bearing or postmenopausal
Anaemia, with lax abdomen
PV: Laxitiy of perineum with bulging and protrusion of mass outside vagina
The parts coming out can be palpated

SAQ 15 What are the complications of prolapse?

- Invalidism
- Cystitis
- Hydronephrosis, hydroureter, renal failure
- Decubitus ulcer
- Pelvic sepsis

SAQ 16 How to prevent prolapse?

Antenatal care with episiotomy during labour, reducing weight, constipation, cough and dysentery.

LAQ 17 What are the treatment of genital prolapse?

The different types of treatments are:

Surgery

Pelvic floor repair (PFR)

- Anterior colporrhaphy for cystocele.
- Posterior colpoperineorrhaphy for rectocele.
- Fothergill operation preserving uterus for uterine prolapse.
- Ward Mayo's operation vaginal hysterectomy with PFR.
- Le Fort's operation vaginal canal partly obliterated in old woman.
- Repair of vault prolapse.
- Repair of urethrocele.

Pessary

- Ring pessary.
- Cup and stem Napier pessary.

Physiotherapy

- Rest.
- Correct retroversion and anaemia.
- Pelvic floor muscle exercise.
- Kegal perineometer exercise.

SAQ 18 What is relaxed perineum?

When vaginal introitus gaps due to relaxation of gynaecological perineum. Treated with operation, or physiotherapy. If in old age and asymptomatic may left untreated.

SAQ 19 What is hypertrophic elongation of cervix?

When the length and breadth of cervix enlarges.

SAQ 20 What is vaginal vault prolapse?

Enterocele, uterovaginal prolapse and vaginal vault prolapse after hysterectomy (abdomen and vagina) together produces vaginal vault prolapse.

SAQ 21 What are the types of hypertrophic elongation of cervix?

It may enlarge in: (i) vaginal portion and (ii) supravaginal portion.

SAQ 22 How to diagnose hypertrophic elongation of cervix?

(i) History of something coming down P/V. Leucorrhoea if chronic cervicitis.
(ii) P/V inspection – cervix outside vagina,
Palpation – Vaginal fornices are deeper and elongated confirmed by uterine sound and hysterography.

SAQ 23 How to treat hypertrophic elongation of cervix?

Surgery for partial amputation of vaginal cervix.

27 Infertility; Vaginismus; Dyspareunia, Frigidity

SAQ 1 Define infertility.

Infertility or sterility means inability by a female to conceive after one year of sexual life without contraceptive intervention.

SAQ 2 What are the causes of infertility?

The infertility may arise of fault in production or conduction of ovum or sperm or fault in performance of coitus.

LAQ 3 What are the factors involved in the process of infertility?

It may be physiological (before puberty or menopause) or pathological.

Faults in male partner

Age over 45, smoking, diabetes, hypopituitary, hypothyroid, adrenal disorders, nervousness, hydrocele, Klinefelter's syndrome, mumps, varicocele, epididymis urethritis, phimosis.

Faults in female partner

PT; anaemia, tubal spasm, vaginismus, vaginal stenosis, cervical hypoplasia or neoplasia or infection fibroid uterus, salpingitis, oophoritis, ovarian tumour

Maladjustment between husband and wife; agglutination of sperms

SAQ 4 What is primary and secondary infertility?

In primary infertility, conception has never occurred and in secondary infertility, conception has failed to take place after a period of fertility.

SAQ 5 What are the causes of secondary infertility?

For male

Age, diabetes, obesity, hydrocele, vasectomy, endocrine diseases (hypopituitary; hypothyroid), etc.

For female

Age, obesity, vaginal stenosis, prolapse, TB of endometrium, cornial block, PID, IUCD, ovarian tumour, tubectomy, Stein-Leventhal syndrome, Sheehan's syndrome, etc.

LAQ 6 How to investigate in a case of infertility?

Both the partners should be interviewed and investigated for relevant reasons.

(i) Clinical history: Age, history of illness, local exam of genitalia

(ii) General survey of husband and wife

(iii) Clinical investigation of wife: Age, occupation, present history, menstrual history, obstetric history for secondary infertility. Marital history, past history personal history, pelvic examination.

Inestigations:

In male

- Semen analysis
- Blood group; VDRL PPBS; urinalysis; 17 ketosteroids; PBI; T3; T4; TSH.
- Testicular biopsy.
- Vasography.
- Sperm autoagglutination.

In female

- Tubal insufflation Rubin test
- Hysterosalpingography
- Laparoscopy with dye instillation.

Ovulation test by

- Basal body temperature
- Endometrial histology
- Evaluation for ova.

Test for cervical mucus

- Postcoital test.
- Fern test.
- Spinnbarkeit cervical mucus thread test.
- Incompatibility test.
- Luteal phase adequacy.

Endocrine assay for
Oestrogen, progesterone T_3 T_4; TSH; PBI; gonadotrophin, urinary 17 ketosteroids.
VDRL; CXR(PA) PPBS; Hb%, vaginal discharge, blood groups, etc.

SAQ 7 What is fern test?

Under the influence of oestrogen fern pattern of cervical mucus can be visualized under microscope from 5–6 days with maximum before ovulation. If it persists up to 22 days of period suggest anovulation. It results from crystallization of NaCl due to oestrogen effect.

SAQ 8 What is spinnbarkeit cervical mucus thread test?

Ovulation has got great elasticity on cervical mucus which can be stretchable up to 6 cm due to oestrogen activity.

SAQ 9 What is vaginismus?

Here there is spasmodic contraction of pelvic muscles often associated with gluteal muscles and abductor muscles of thigh when coitus or vaginal examination is tried.

SAQ 10 What is dyspareunia?

When the coitus is painful.

SAQ 11 What are the causes of dyspareunia?

In male

Psychological, obesity, impotence, phimosis, hypospadias, penile sore, IUCD thread.

In female

Obesity, abortion, tight hymen, vaginal atrophy, postmenopausal virilism, OCP. Haemorrhoids, endometriosis, retroversion, TO mass, bartholinitis, repair of episiotomy.

SAQ 12 How to treat narrow vaginal introitus with rigid hymen?

By Fentons operation where under GA, a transverse incision is made at mucocutaneous junction of fourchette and flap of posterior vaginal mucosa is dissected of perineal muscle up to hymeneal ring. Hymeneal ring is dissected, perineal muscle divided and vaginal flaps margins are transversely sutured.

SAQ 13 What is frigidity?

Lack of libido.

SAQ 14 What are the causes of premature ejaculation?

- Infrequent coitus
- Overexcitement
- Coitus attempted before strong erection.

28 Fertility Control

LAQ 1 What is fertility? What are the factors determine fertility?

Fertility means actual bearing of children. Some demographers prefer the word natality for fertility.

Following factors determine fertility:

1. Age of marriage
2. Duration of married life
3. Spacing of children
4. Education
5. Caste and religion
6. Economic status and nutrition
7. Adoption of family planning services.

LAQ 2 What is family planning? What are its objectives?

It is a way of thinking and living which is adopted voluntarily, upon the basis of knowledge, attitude and responsible decisions by individuals and couples in order to promote the health and welfare of the family group to contribute effectively to the social development of a country.

It is aimed at:

- To avoid unwanted birth
- To bring wanted birth
- To regulate intervals of pregnancies
- To control the time at which birth occurs in relation to the ages of patient
- To determine numbers of children in family.

SAQ 3 What is new revised population policy?

- Advancing age of marriage of girls to 20
- Promoting 2 children norm
- Increasing female literacy
- Increasing demand for contraception and spacing method
- Increasing child survival by universal immunizations
- Linkage between antipoverty scheme and involving non-governmental agencies to improve family planning infrastructure.

SAQ 4 What is the principle of rhythm methods and how safe period is calculated?

Abstinence during fertile period.

Here duration of 12 menstrual cycles are obtained. The unsafe day is obtained by deducting 18 from the shortest cycle and 11 from the longest cycle, e.g. if shortest cycle is 25 and longest cycle is 30 then 25–18 = 7 days and 30–11 = 19 days. Thus abstinence from 7 to 19 days are suggested, charts are available.

LAQ 5 What are the different contraceptive methods?

The different contraceptive methods are:

Temporary methods

Without any contrivance

- Coitus interruptus.
- Rhythm method.

With contrivance

A. Physical method.
   Conventional – condom.
   Vaginal diaphragm; condom bikini.
B. Chemical methods.
   i. Foam – tablets; aerosol.
   ii. Cream, jellies, paste.
   iii. Suppositories.
   iv. Soluble film – C-film inserted manually.
C. IUCD.
D. Oral contraceptive.

Permanent methods

1. Tubectomy.
2. Vasectomy.

SAQ 6 What are the advantages and disadvantages of rhythm method?

Advantages: Simple, safe, always available, acceptable.

Disadvantages: Cost of calendar, 35% effective, psychological effect.

SAQ 7 What are the advantages and disadvantages of coitus interruptus?

Advantages: Simple, safe, cheap, available, acceptable

Disadvantages: Sexual pleasure hampered, 35% effective, psychological effect, decision making is important.

SAQ 8 What are the advantages and disadvantages of condom?

Advantages: Simple, safe, protects STD, widely used.

Disadvantages: Allergic; hampers sexual pleasure.

SAQ 9 Name some vaginal diaphragms.

Dutch cap, Vault cap, Cervical cap, Vimule cap.

SAQ 10 How many condoms are required per year to protect a couple?

72.

SAQ 11 What are the disadvantages of vaginal diaphragm?

Though it has no systemic side effects, it has following disadvantages: Needs motivation, training, costly, privacy for insertion and removal, not very effective.

SAQ 12 What are the advantages and disadvantages of chemical contraception?

Advantages: Safe, simple.

Disadvantages: May be irritating, low effective, cost factor, less acceptable.

SAQ 13 Name some chemical contraceptives.

They are chemical barriers to sperm and kill them, viz.

Jelly	Cream and paste	Suppositories	Foam tab.	Aerosol foam	Soluble film
Orthogynol Ortho-Preceptin gel.	Delfen.	Rendells.	Contabs.	Delfen foam. EMCO foam.	C-film.

LAQ 14 What is IUCD?

These are plastic intrauterine devices for contraception, viz.

Unmedicated

- Margulies spiral
- Lippes loop
- Figure of eight plastic Birabnrg bow
- Soonawala
- Plastic with magnetic strip (Antigon F)
- Saf T coil
- Hall stone ring (nylon made).
- Dalkon shield
- Ota ring

Medicated

- Copper – T
- Copper – 7
- Multiload copper-250, 375
- Progestasert (progesterone discharging T device).
- T cu 380A or Ag

SAQ 15 Who is the ideal candidate of IUCD?

- Has one child
- No PID
- Regular period
- Willing to see IUD tail
- Monogamous relation
- Can come for follow up

SAQ 16 What are the advantages of copper devices?

- Low expulsion and side effects (pain; bleeding)
- Better tolerated with increased effectiveness
- Effective as postcoital contraceptive if inserted with 3–5 days of unprotected pregnancy

SAQ 17 What is the mechanism of action of IUCD?

Foreign body reaction causing cellular and biochemical change in uterine fluid impairing viability of gametes to fertilize and prevent implant by inhibiting zinc containing enzyme carbonic anhydrase.

SAQ 18 When to insert IUCD?

Within a week of menstruation and 6 weeks of postpartum period.

SAQ 19 How long IUCD should be kept?

If asymptomatic then indefinitely. But ICMR recommend 8 years. It should be changed 2–3 years to prevent embedded in endometrium. Copper T200 is effective for 3 years.

SAQ 20 What are the contraindications of IUCD?

Contraindications

Relative

- Anaemia
- Menorrhagia
- PID
- Congenital uterial defect
- Fibroid

Absolute

- Pregnancy
- PID
- Undiagnosed bleeding P/V
- Ca cervix and uterus
- Ectopic pregnancy

SAQ 21 What are the advantages and disadvantages of IUCD?

Advantages: Reversable, no side effects, cost-effective, acceptable.
Disadvantages: Need supervision and expert for insertion, side effect needs removal.

SAQ 22 What are the complications and side effects of IUCD?

- Bleeding
- Pain
- Pelvic infection
- Uterine perforation
- Pregnancy
- Ectopic pregnancy
- Expulsion
- Fertility after removal, cancer and teratogenicity
- Rarely mortality.

SAQ 23 Classify hormonal contraceptives.

Oral

- Combined pill
- Progesterone only pill
- Postcoital pill
- Once a month (long acting pill)
- Sequential pill
- Male pill

Slow release depot formulation

- Injectable
- Subcutaneous implants
- Vaginal ring

SAQ 24 What do you mean by: (i) Combined pills, (ii) Mini-pills, (iii) Sequential pills, (iv) Phased regimen, (v) Post-coital pills?

(i) **Combined pills:** Contain oestrogen and progesterone.

(ii) **Mini-pills:** Contain low dose progesterone only.

(iii) **Sequential pills:** Contain oestrogen in 1st 15th day, then progesterone for 15 days.

(iv) **Phased regimen:** Dose of oestrogen is kept constant progesterone in low in 1st phase and gradually higher in 2nd and third phase.

(v) **Post-coital pills (Yuzpe method):** Used for unprotected pregnancy, contain levonorgestrol 0.5 + ethinyl/oestradiol 0.1 mg (ovaral 2 tab) taken within 72 hours preferably 12 hours.

SAQ 25 How does OCP act?

- Postcoital pill inhibits implantation.
- Modify uterine and tubular contraction unfavourable for fertilization.
- Progesterone makes cervical secretion thick and hostile for sperm penetration.
- Reinforce normal feedback inhibition of gonadotropin release by progesterone to inhibit ovulation.

SAQ 26 How does male pill acts?

The search for male pill going on. It probably acts by preventing spermatogenesis, interfering sperm maturation and storage and transport, altering constituents of seminal fluid.

Gossypol obtained from cotton seeds produces azoospermia and oligospermia.

LAQ 27 Mention some adverse effects of OCP.

No serious side effects

Nausea, vomiting, morning sickness, headache migraine, breast discomfort, break through bleeding.

Serious complications

Leg, pulmonary vein cerebral or coronary vessels thrombosis, genital carcinoma, hepatoma, gallstone.

Late side effects

Thrombosis, weight gain, chloasma, pruritus vulvae, mood swinging, Carbohydrate intolerance

LAQ 28 What are the contraindications of OCP?

Contraindications

Relative contraindications

- Diabetes
- Obesity
- Smoking
- Undiagnosed
- Vaginal bleeding
- Fibroid
- Age above 35
- Mentally ill
- Migraine
- Gallstone
- Hypertension.

Absolute contraindications

- Thromboembolism
- Hypertension
- Hyperlipidemia
- Liver disease and jaundice
- Porphyria
- Suspected malignancy
- Before surgery

SAQ 29 How to chose hormonal pills?

Women with premenstrual tension, headache, menorrhagia, i.e. oestrogenic effects are given progesterone pill.

Women showing scanty mens, leg cramps, acne, dry vagina, fullness of breast, i.e. progesterone effect given low dose progesterone.

In some countries, oral pills with low doses are started.

SAQ 30 What are the other effects of OCP?

(i) Lower chances of endometrial and ovarian cancer, (ii) prevents anaemia by lowering menstrual loss, (iii) improved PID and endometriosis, (iv) reduces incidence of fibrocystic breast disease.

SAQ 31 What is centchroman?

Non-steroidal oestrogen antagonist developed by CDRI act as anti-implantation with long $^t/_2$, given 30 mg, biweekly for 3 months and then weekly (marketed as Saheli or Centron.)

SAQ 32 Name some injectable contraceptives.

(i) Depot medroxy progesterone acetate (DMPA) 150–400 mg. At 3–6 months interval.
(ii) Norethinidrone enanthate (NEE) 200 mg at 2–3 months interval.

SAQ 33 What are the guidelines, for terminal method of sterilization?

- Age of the husband should be more than 25 and less than 50 years
- Couple should have 2 living children
- If couple has three children, lower limit may be relaxed.

SAQ 34 What are the advantages and disadvantages of vasectomy?

Advantages: Simple, safe, low cost, effective.
Disadvantages: Permanent, irreversible and side effects of haematoma, granuloma, infection, sperm antibodies.

SAQ 35 What postoperative advice should be given to vasectomy patients?

- 30 ejaculation requires for seminal examination negative, should use condoms
- To avoid bath for 24 hours and cycling and weight lifting for 15 days
- Stitches to be removed on 5–7 days.

SAQ 36 What are the different methods for female sterilization?

Minilaparotomy or laparoscopy.

SAQ 37 What are the advantages and disadvantages of female sterilization?

Advantages: Safe, low failure, acceptable, no change in health.

Disadvantages: Irreversible, hospital procedure, costlier than vasectomy.

SAQ 38 How to suggest family welfare method to acceptor?

All methods are described to acceptor and it is cafeteria choice.

SAQ 39 What is birth control vaccine?

It is immunization with vaccine prepared from beta subunits of HCG which block continuation of pregnancy. Antibodies appear in 4–6 weeks and declines in 6–11 months.

SAQ 40 How to evaluate contraceptive method?

It is expressed as failure rate per hundred woman years of exposure or Pearl index.

$$\text{Failure rate per HWY} = \frac{\text{Total accidental pregnancies}}{\text{Total months of exposure}} \times 1200$$

Diagnosis of Sex; Intersex, Virilism, Hirsutism

29

SAQ 1 How the diagnosis of sex is made?

It is done by following methods:

- Morphology
  - Sex chromatin
  - Gondadal structure
  - Internal genitalia
  - External genitalia
  - Hormones
- Gender role or psychosexual behavior

SAQ 2 What is sex chromatin?

The number of barr body or sex chromatin in a nucleus is one less than number of X chromosomes, In sex chromosomal anomaly, seen in buccal smear in over 25% of females.

SAQ 3 What is intersex?

This is individual with anomalous sexual development.

SAQ 4 What is hirsutism?

Abnormal hair growth due to hyperandrogenism in female.

LAQ 5 Classify intersexuality.

It may be as follows:

- At chromosomal level
  - Turner's syndrome.
  - Multiple X syndrome.
  - Klinefelter's syndrome.
- At gonadal level
  - True hermaphrodite.
- Female pseudo-hermaphrodite
  - Drug induced malculinization.
  - Congenital adrenal hyperplasia.
- Male pseudoherma-phrodite
  - Feminizing testicular syndrome.
  - Masculinizing male pseudohermaphrodite.

SAQ 6 What are the causes of hirsutism?

- Genetic
- Physiologic (puberty, pregnancy)
- Iatrogenic (anabolic steroids, streptomycin, dilantin)
- Endocrine: anorexia, nervosa, Cushing's syndrome, acromegaly; adrenogenital syndrome
- Polycystic ovary syndrome
- Brenner's syndrome
- Arrhenoblastoma
- Intersex: Male pseudohermaphrodite.

SAQ 7 What is virilism?

When excess androgen stimulates hair, external genitalia, larynx, and muscle occurs in female is called virilism.

LAQ 8 What are the causes of virilism?

The important causes of virilism are:

Endocrinal

1. **Adrenal diseases**
   - Adrenogenital syndrome
   - Cushing's syndrome
2. Ovarian causes
   - Arrhenoblastoma
   - Stein-Leventhal syndrome
3. Intersex
   - Hermaphrodite (true and male pseudo)
4. Oophorectomy
5. Pituitary
   - Acromegaly
   - Cushing's syndrome
6. Iatrogenic.
   - Anabolic steroids
   - Progesterone OCP
   - Corticosteroids therapy

Genetic

- Familiar and racial

Psychiatric

- Homosexuality
- Transvestism
- Trans-sexuality (urge of woman to change sex)

30 Complete Perineal Tear, Uterine Inversion; RVF

SAQ 1 What is complete perineal tear (CPT)?

It is perineal tear up to sphincter ani externus. It becomes old after three months of delivery.

SAQ 2 What are the causes of CPT?

(i) Obstetric injury (forceps delivery, occipitoposterior, precipitate labour).
(ii) Trauma (fall, piles and fistula operation).

SAQ 3 What are the clinical features of CPT?

Important symptoms and signs are:

Symptoms

- Young with history of difficult delivery
- Stool incontinence

Signs

- Absent perineum
- Absent radial cutaneous rugosites of anus
- Loss of muscle tone of anal canal

SAQ 4 How to treat CPT?

If not treated after delivery, it should be treated after 3 months by operation. Perineorrhaphy operation (Layer's method) or Warren flap method of repair.

SAQ 5 What is inversion of uterus?

It is inside out turning of uterus.

SAQ 6 What are the different operations performed for inversion of uterus?

(i) Haultain's operation (by abdominal route).
(ii) Spinell's operation (by vaginal route).
(iii) Kustner's operation (by vaginal route).

SAQ 7 What is rectovaginal fistula?

Fistulous connection between vagina and rectum abbreviated as RVF. May be in lower, middle or upper third of vagina.

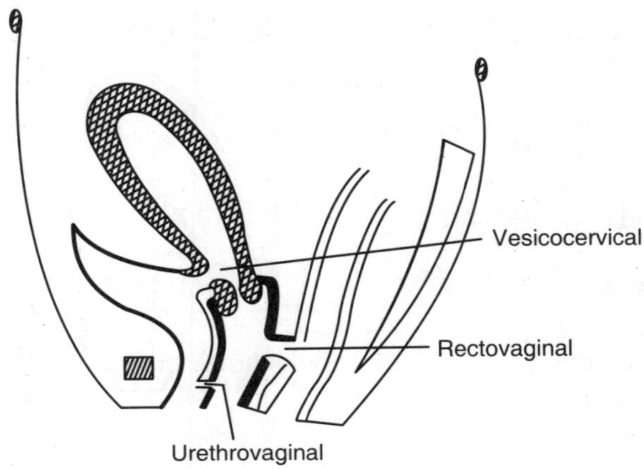

SAQ 8 What are the causes of RVF?

The causes are as follows:

Congenital

- Vestibular anus

Acquired

- Trauma during labour
- Operation
- Pelvic abscess
- Radiation
- Forgotten pessary

SAQ 9 What are the important clinical feature of RVF?

Faecal vaginal discharge. Opening can be seen on posterior vaginal wall on speculum inspection.

SAQ 10 How to treat RVF?

(i) By surgical repairing
(ii) Vestibular anus by Rizzoli's operation
(iii) Colostomy as palliative measure in malignant RVF.

Urinary Incontinence and Genitourinary Fistula

31

SAQ 1 What is urinary incontinence? What are their types?

Involuntary urinary leakage is called urinary incontinence. It may be of following types:

True incontinence	Urge incontinence	Stress incontinence	Overflow incontinence

- Due to developmental defect.
- Overstretching.
- Genitourinary fistula.

SAQ 2 What is stress incontinence?

Urine leaks unconsciously in female when intra-abdominal pressure rises. Causes are:

- Postpartum
- Postmenopausal
- Postoperative
- Developmental.

SAQ 3 How to treat stress incontinence?

(i) Physiotherapy.

(ii) Operation – initially utrethroplasty or Kelly's operation followed by:
  - Vasicourethral suspension
  - Sling operation (by Aldridge or Millin operation)

SAQ 4 What is urge incontinence?

Here there is urgent desire to void urine with large volume of urine leaks when bladder is full, before the patient reaching the toilet.

SAQ 5 What are the causes of urge incontinence?

Nervous system diseases

- Disseminated sclerosis
- Neurosis
- CVA

Local pelvic causes

- Cystitis (UTI; TB)
- Pelvic tumours
- Hunner's ulcer

SAQ 6 What is dysuria?

When pain is felt during or after micturition.

SAQ 7 What are the causes of dysuria?

Dysuria

Vulval lesions

- Inflammation
- Carcinoma of vulvae
- Kraurosis vulvae

Bladder causes

- Cystitis
- Following catheterization
- Stone in bladder
- Radiation cystitis
- Growth in bladder
- Cystourethrocele

Urethral causes

- Caruncle
- Inflammation
- Carcinoma of meatus
- Honeymoon cystitis (trauma to urethra and bladder)

SAQ 8 What is urethral caruncle?

It is swelling of mucosa in posterior lip of external urinary meatus.

SAQ 9 How to treat urethral caruncle?

Excision of caruncle followed by sutured and cauterisation of raw area. Histology of excision tissue should be done.

SAQ 10 What are the clinical features of urethral caruncle?

Symptoms

- Dysuria
- Irregular bleeding P/V
- Urinary retention
- Dyspareunia
- Asymptomatic

Signs

Painful red pea-like protruding mass on posterior lip of external urethral meatus, which bleeds on touching

SAQ 11 What are the causes, of retention of urine in female?

Retention of urine in female may be due to:

Medical causes

- Hysteria
- Tabes dorsalis
- Spinal injury

Local causes

Gynaecological

- Fibroid
- Ovarian tumour
- Pessary
- Retroverted gravid uterus
- Ca vagina cervix
- Pelvic hematocele

Postoperative

- Sling operation

Urethrovesicle

- Urethral caruncle
- Diverticulum
- Cystocele
- Bladder stone or stricture

SAQ 12 What is vesico-vaginal fistula (VVF)?

It is the fistulous communication between urinary bladder and upper half of anterior vagina may be as small as pins head to 1" through which bladder mucosa may prolapse.

SAQ 13 What are the causes of VVF?

(i) Obstetrical trauma (obstructed labour, or obstetric operations)
(ii) Trauma
(iii) Gynaecological operation (colporrhaphy, hysterectomy)
(iv) Cancer (cervix, vagina or bladder)
(v) Inflammation
(vi) Congenital
(vii) Overdose of radiation

LAQ 14 What are the clinical features of VVF?

Clinical features of VVF are as follows:

Symptoms

- Dribbling urine P/V and inability to pass urine through normal orifice.

Signs

Short stature, irritable wet clothing and perineum. Vaginal examination may show the fistula, catheter may come out of fistula and fistula can be palpated P/R may show CPT and RVF. Dye test, swab test, cystoscopy may demonstrate the fistula.

LAQ 15 How to treat VVF?

Small fistula may heal spontaneously in 1–2 months by conservative treatment. The healing may hasten with catheterization (for 10–14 days); antibiotics; semiprone position and alkali mixture.

Surgical repair of VVF is treatment of choice, by

- Vaginal approach
- Transvesicle approach
- Transperitoneal approach

- Sims edge paring (saucerization)
- Flap splitting method.

The locally irrepairable VVF requires urinary diversion operation by.

Ureterocolic anastomosis by
- → Coffey's method.
- → Nesbit's method.
- → Leadbetter method.

But these anastomosis operation may produce:

- Kidney failure
- Hydronephrosis
- Ascending urinary infection
- Hyperchloremic acidosis due absorption of NaCl and K loss from lower lumen.

SAQ 16 What are the symptoms and treatment of urethrovaginal fistula?

May be symptomless or urinary dribbling on medial aspect of thigh. Treated by constructing new urethra.

SAQ 17 How to treat vasicocervical fistula?

By local repair.

SAQ 18 How to treat VVF of cancer or post-radiation?

Prognostically bad. Following operations are performed.

(i) Ureterocolic anastomosis.
(ii) Latzko's colpocleisis (closure of vagina below fistula).

SAQ 19 How to treat rectovaginal fistula and vesicovaginal fistula if occurs in combination?

Both fistulas should be tried to repair in single sitting if possible. VVF is repaired first than left inguinal colostomy, then repair RVF and close colostomy.

If local repair of either fistula is not possible then partial closure of vagina (colpocleisis) may be performed. If VVF is not repairable, the RVF is repaired followed by ureterocolic anastomosis.

32 Pelvic Inflammatory Diseases

SAQ 1 What are the common causes of genital tract infection?

(i) Pyogenic
(ii) Tubercular
(iii) STD
(iv) Parasitic
(v) Fungal

The infection may occur in upper and lower genital tract by direct spread, venous spread, lymphatic spread, haematogenous spread and by continuity.

SAQ 2 What are the etiologies of acute cervicitis? How is it treated?

Gonorrhea, pyogenic infection after abortion or childbirth, acute on chronic cervicitis.
Treatment: Bed rest, antibiotics are treatment. No vaginal douching should be given.

SAQ 3 What are the etiologies of acute endometritis?

The etiologies of acute endometritis and metritis are:
(i) Puerperal or postabortal infection
(ii) Gynaecological operation/IUCD or D/C
(iii) Gonorrhoea
(iv) Polyp
(v) Fibroid
(vi) Carcinoma

LAQ 4 What is acute salpingitis? Describe its etiology, clinical features and treatment?

Inflammation of fallopian tube may be bilateral or unilateral due to:
(i) Gonococcal
(ii) Pyogenic
(iii) Postpartum or abortal or surgical
(iv) From infected cervix, appendix

(v) Tubercular. It may:
- Resolutes
- Or may produce hydrosalpinx
- TO mass
- Pelvic abscess.

Clinical features, H/o recent delivery, abortion, operation, IUCD.

Symptoms

Fever, vomiting, pain abdomen, irregular period, vaginal discharge.

Signs

Toxemia, tachycardia, purulent discharge P/V with tenderness, abdominal rigidity.

Leukocytosis and C/S for cervical smear examination.

Treatment: Rest in semirecumbent position, suitable autibiotics. Drainage of pelvic abscess by posterior colpotomy.

SAQ 5 What is perimetritis and parametritis?

Perimetritis (acute pelvic peritonitis) is inflammation of the pelvic peritoneum.
Parametritis (acute pelvic cellulitis) is inflammation of paracervical mass, i.e. parametrium.

SAQ 6 Define pelvic abscess.

It is defined as collection of pus in the pelvis in pouch of Douglas. It may be intraperitoneal or parametrial.

SAQ 7 What are the causes of pelvic abscess?

Microbial infection due to:

Pelvic causes

Puerperal or postabortal, peri- or parametritis, infected pelvic haematocele, ovarian cyst or fibroid, surgery (tubectomy or hysterectomy).

Extrapelvic causes

Abscess in surrounding hollow viscous

SAQ 8 How to investigate pelvic abscess?

(i) History
(ii) Clinical features—tender lower abdomen, fluctuant elastic tenderness on posterior fornix and front of rectum. Leukocytosis and needling of pouch of Douglas reveals pus.

SAQ 9 Define chronic cervicitis. What are their types?

It is defined as localized chronic inflammatory lesion of the surrounding fibromuscular structure of cervix generally associated with cervical erosion.

Types: (i) Chronic endocervicitis with mucous, (ii) cervical erosion, (iii) hypertrophy elongation of cervix.

Microscopically: Round cell infiltration around endocervical glands of cervical stroma.

SAQ 10 What is cervical erosion?

It is generally a disease of reproductive age group characterized by reddened area of portiovaginalis around external os, where the stratified squamous epithelium is replaced by columnar epithelium of the endocervix.

It may of following types:

Congenital

Lasting few days due to maternal oestrogen.

Acquired

- Simple flat type
- Papillary type
- Follicular type

SAQ 11 How to treat cervical erosion?

The congenital, pregnancy, erosion of virgin, OCP induced erosion does not require treatment. Symptomatic erosion treated by:

- Diathermy or electrocautery 5–7 days after menstrual cesation.
- Conisation.
- Surgery (partial amputation of cervix or tracheorrhaphy).
- Cryosurgery.

In all the cervical erosions, patient cytology diagnosis should be routinally performed.

SAQ 12 What are the contraindications of electrocautery in cervical erosion?

- Acute cervicitis.
- Suspicious malignancy.
- Acute pelvic inflammation.

SAQ 13 How to treat cervical erosion in virgins?

In virgin, the cervical erosion is mostly due to gonococcal, trichomonal or tuberculosis. It should be treated plus correction of menstrual disorder, anaemia and general health.

SAQ 14 What are the signs and symptoms of chronic metritis?

It may be due to acute metritis, tubercular metritis symptomatized by backache, congestive dysmenorrhoea, menorrhagia. Uterus enlarges with adnexal inflammation.

SAQ 15 What is chronic endometritis? How to treat it?

Chronic endometritis are of following types:

(i) Senile endometritis (with thin foul smelling vaginal discharge, may be blood stained).
(ii) Chronic interstitial endometritis due to IUCD, neoplasm or retained placental bits.

Treatment:

- Malignancy should be ruled out
- D/C if pyometra
- Antibiotics

SAQ 16 Define chronic salpingitis and oophoritis.

Generally, chronic inflammation of fallopian tube and ovary occurs together producing TO mass. It generally occurs as a consequence of pelvic inflammation. Pathological lesions are:

- Hydrosalpinx
- Pyosalpinx
- Chronic interstitial salpingitis
- Salpingitis istmica nodosa.
- Chronic oophoritis

SAQ 17 What are the varieties of chronic oophoritis?

It may be:

- Chronic interstitial diphtheritis
- Chroni perioophoritis.
- Ovarian abscess.
- Generally, it occurs as a consequence of inflammation of fallopian tubes.

LAQ 18 How the chronic salpingo-oophoritis patient presents?

Presentation of salpingo-oophoritis.

Symptoms

- Backache
- Vague pain of lower abdomen
- Menstrual disorders (menorrhagia, congestive dysmenorrhoea)
- Sterility
- Dysuria and painful defecation
- Fever
- Dyspareunia

Signs

General health poor, anaemia P/A: Hydrosalpinx and pyosalpinx can be felt over inguinal canal. P/V lateral fornices may feel hydro- or pyosalpinx. Uterus may retroverted.

SAQ 19 Describe in brief the pathology of genital tuberculosis.

Tuberculosis can affect any genital organ mostly secondary rarely primary. Generally secondary may spread to genital organ from PT by: (i) direct through peritoneum, (ii) blood or lymphatics. The sites involved are fallopian tube, corpus uteri (endometritis), cervix or ovaries.

SAQ 20 How to treat chronic salpingitis and oophoritis?

Treatment of salpingitis and oophoritis

Conservative

- Treat sepsis with suitable antibiotics.
- Anti-inflammatory.
- Correct anaemia.

Surgery

- Remove hydrosalpinx pyosalpinx by laparotomy.
- Elderly women with complete family, total hysterectomy with removal of bilateral adenexal mass.

LAQ 21 What are the clinical features of genital tuberculosis?

Clinical features of genital tuberculosis

Symptoms

Infertility, menstrual disorder (amenorrhoea menorrhagia), pelvic pain. No symptoms.

Signs

Anaemia, poor general health, P/A tubes may be enlarged above inguinal ligament P/V bilateral fixed mass may be felt on lateral fornix, the same may be felt P/R.

SAQ 22 What is tubo-ovarian mass?

When the chronic inflammation of fallopian tubes, ovary produces adherence with each other to produce a mass, generally bilateral. The types of lesion may be hydrosalpinx and pyosalpinx adherent to tubo-ovarian cyst, tubo-ovarian abscess, chronic interstitial salpingo-oophoritis.

LAQ 23 Name the condition when mass can be felt in pouch of Douglas.

Mass in pouch of Douglas

Congenital

- Ectopic kidney
- Rudimentary uterine horn

Pathological

Inflammatory TO mass; TO cyst, appendicular lump. Fluid (haematocele, pelvic abscess; ascitis, neoplastic, foreign body.)

Physiological

Retroverted gravid uterus, impacted faces in rectum; abdominal pregnancy, loop of intestine.

SAQ 24 What are the causes of vaginitis?

VAGINITIS

Bacterial

- Gonococcal
- Tubercular
- Syphilitic
- Lymphogranuloma inguinale

Parasitic

- Schistosomiasis
- Amoebiasis
- Oxyriasis
- Trichomoniasis

Fungal

- Monilial
- Foreign body
- Douches
- Prolapse

Nonspecific

- Pessary

SAQ 25 What are the signs and symptoms of *Trichomonas vaginalis*?

Symptoms

- Vaginal discharge
- Itching vulva
- Dyspareunia
- Dysuria.

Signs

Vagina red swellen and tender, bleed on touching the red papillae with copious greenish yellow frothy offensive discharge, cervix red with or without erosion.

SAQ 26 How to treat trichomoniasis?

Orally: Metronidazole or tinidazole.
Vaginally: Floraquin or intestopan vaginal tablets.

LAQ 27 What are the symptoms and signs and senile vaginitis and its treatment?

Atrophic vaginal epithelium with non-specific inflammation, patchy ulceration on vaginal wall occurs in senile vaginitis with the following clinical features.

Symptoms

- Blood stained yellow vaginal discharge with itching of introitus
- Dyspareunia
- Dysuria

Signs

- Minute punctate red ulceration with adhesion
- Vault contraction

Treatment orally ethanyl oestradiol 0.05 mg OD for two weeks in hysterectomised patient. Locally cleanliness, lactic and ½% vaginal douche or dienosterol or hydrocortisone cream locally.

SAQ 28 What is vulvitis?

Inflammation of vulva. It may be:

Acute

- Gonococcal or pyococcal
- Trichomonial
- Diabetic
- Monilial

Chronic

- Leprosy
- Filariasis
- Syphilis
- Tuberculosis

LAQ 29 Describe the pathology of gonorrhoea of female genitalia.

Caused by *N. gonorrhoeae*, may present as acute or chronic.

Acute gonorrhoea

Lower genital tract

- Vulvitis
- Vaginitis
- Bartholinitis
- Cystitis
- Trigonitis

Upper genital tract

- Cervicitis
- Salpingitis
- Oophoritis
- Peritonitis

Chronic gonorrhoea

May involve cervix, urethra, Bartholin's gland.

Other sites of genital tract: Urethra, bladder, anus, rectum, joint, conjunctiva and septicaemia may be involved.

33 Uterine Fibroid and Endometriosis

SAQ 1 What is uterine fibroid?

It is benign growth from muscular layer of uterus. Its appropriate terminology is fibromyoma or myoma of uterus. Histologically, consisting of mature and immature muscles of uterus.

SAQ 2 Name of the sites where uterine fibroid generally occurs.

Mostly in body of uterus or rarely cervix.

SAQ 3 What are the different types of fibroid?

(i) Intramural (interstitial)
(ii) Subserous
(iii) Submucous

SAQ 4 What are the fate of submucous fibroid?

(i) Polyp formation
(ii) Infection
(iii) Turn malignant
(iv) Inversion of uterus

SAQ 5 How the uterine fibroid looks like in naked eye?

Single or multiple, with varying size, spherical, firmer than uterus. Cut surfaces are pale, white, whorl-like trabeculation, with pseudocapsular layer with loose areolar tissue separating the surrounding muscle tumour bulges out. Center of fibroid is less vascular.

SAQ 6 What changes can take place in uterine fibroid?

- Hyaline degeneration
- Cystic degeneration
- Fatty degeneration

- Calcification
- Red degeneration
- Necrosis
- Infection
- Atrophic degeneration
- Malignant changes (sarcoma)
- Angioma
- Lymphangiectasis

SAQ 7 What are the clinical features of uterine fibroid?

Clinical features of fibroid

Symptoms

May be symptomless or menorrhagia, dysmenorrhoea, abdominal lump, white discharge, pain; infertility, symptoms of anaemia.

Signs

Anaemia P/R, P/A and P/V shows lump.

SAQ 8 What are the causes of menorrhagia in fibroid?

- Increase of endometrial surface
- Increased vascularity
- Fibroid impairing haemostasis
- Hyperplasia of endometrium.

SAQ 9 What are the causes of death in uterine fibroid if left untreated?

- Haemorrhage
- Anaemia
- Peritonitis
- Sarcoma
- Intraperitoneal haemorrhage

LAQ 10 What is the principles of the treatment of uterine fibroid?

Conservative treatment

Surgical treatment

Radiotherapy

Little scope with bad surgical risk, viz. cardiac disease.

Palliative treatment for bleeding

Expectant treatment

Abdominal
- Myomectomy
- Hysterectomy

Vaginal
- Myomectomy
- Hysterectomy

- Haemostasis for bleeding.
- Testosterone propionate 25 mg IM OD × 4 days.

or

- Primolut N 5 mg 1 tab TDS till bleeding stops

or

- Mifepristone

SAQ 11 What are the etiologies of fibroid?

Not definitely known. The probable causes are:
- Heredity
- Oestrogen dependent increased blood supply
- Generally nulliparous
- In reproductive age group

SAQ 12 What location cervical fibroid generally arises?

Portiovaginalis or supravaginal cervix (anterior, posterior, lateral, central).

SAQ 13 How to treat cervical fibroid?

Symptomless requires no treatment. Lage supravaginal fibroid producing symptoms treated operatively by: (a) myomectomy, (b) hysterectomy.

SAQ 14 What is uterine polyp? What are their types?

The pedunculated growth from uterine body or cervix is called uterine polyp. It may be: (i) mucous, (ii) placental, (iii) fibroid or (iv) malignant in types.

SAQ 15 What is sarcoma cervicis botryoides?

The grape-like sarcoma of infancy from either cervix or vagina. Histologically, grape-like sarcoma in infancy shows myxomatous tissue with sarcoma cells with covered epithelium.

LAQ 16 What are the clinical features of malignant uterine polyps?

It generally occurs in childbearing age rarely on menopause. Sarcomatous polyp may arise in infants.

Clinical features

Symptoms

- White discharge
- Metrorrhagia
- Congestive dysmenorrhoea
- Menorrhagia
- Irregular vaginal bleeding in menopausal woman
- Something coming down P/V or retention of urine.

Signs

Polyp can be seen or palpable which is friable and prone to haemorrhage

SAQ 17 What is endometriosis?

It is functional ectopic endometrium, viz.(i) uterine endometriosis or adenomyosis, (ii) extrauterine endometriosis (ovary, peritoneum, laparotomy scar, appendix, bladder, urethra, umbilicus, hernia, fallopian tubes, lungs, pleura).

SAQ 18 What are the different theories of endometriosis for its ectopic location?

- Implantation theory of Sampson.
- Direct extension theory of Cullen.
- Serosal metaplasia theory of Iwanoff.
- Venous dissemination theory of Javert.
- Lymphatic dissemination theory of Halban.

SAQ 19 What is chocolate cyst or tarry cyst or endometrial cyst?

It is ovarian endometriosis producing chocolate coloured cyst of 1½ – 2" in diameter adherent to surrounding structure containing menstrual blood. There may not be endometrial lining, but there is connective tissue, macrophages ingested blood pigments (pseudoxanthoma cells).

SAQ 20 What is adenomyosis?

Endometrial growth within uterine wall locally or diffusely.

SAQ 21 What complications may arise out of endometriosis?

- Ovarian cyst
- Adenocarcinoma
- Intestinal obstruction

SAQ 22 What is the prognosis of endometriosis?

It is benign condition either retrogresses spontaneously or after pregnancy or menopause.

LAQ 23 What are the clinical features of endometriosis?

Occurs in women of reproductive age group (30–50 years). Adenomyosis occurs in parous women, otherwise they are infertile.

CLINICAL FEATURES

Symptoms

Adenomyosis

- Menorrhagia
- Colicky dysmenorrhoea

Endometriosis

- Pelvic pain
- Dysmenorrhoea
- Dyspareunia
- Infertility
- Backache
- Painful nodule with menstruation at different sites
- Pyrexia
- Asymptomatic

Signs

P/A: There may not be any abnormality
P/V: Uterus enlarged and ectopic endometium in pelvis may be palpated.

LAQ 24 How to treat endometriosis?

TREATMENT

Hormone therapy

- Norethisterone acetate (norlestrin) from 5th day to next mens.

or

Primolut – N

or

Danazol 400–800 mg to produce pseudopregnancy.

or

Depoprovera 2 ml every 2 weeks for 4 doses.

Surgery

Extensive

(i) Total hysterectomy with bilateral salpingo-oophorectomy.

(ii) Conservative

(a) Ovarian cyst and pelvic extragenital lesions are excised.

(b) Ventro-suspension and presacral neurectomy. If patients child bearing function to be preserved

Radiotherapy

Used when surgery is contraindicated to produce artificial menopause

SAQ 25 What is Gartner duct cyst?

It is cystic dilatation of Gartner duct, generally on lateral vaginal wall. Treated by excision otherwise infection and suppuration may occur.

SAQ 26 What is vaginal adenosis?

It is non-neoplastic vaginal mucosal change generally found in females born by women treated with diethylstilbesterol in early pregnancy.

SAQ 27 What is Bartholin's cyst?

It is retention cyst of Bartholin's gland or Bartholin's ducts, due to stenosis or calculus, presents with progressive swelling of vulva with difficulty in walking. Treated by excision or marsupialization.

SAQ 28 What is hydradenoma?

It is rare benign tumour of sweat gland at labia majora.

SAQ 29 What is condyloma?

Condyloma (acuminata or lata) is (called venereal wart) papillomatous growth of the vulva arise as pointed warty multiple growth on perineum, vulva or buttocks due to irritation by chronic discharge (veneral or nonveneral).

Treated by local application of podophylin 25% in paraffin or excision or cauterization or cryosurgery.

34 Malignancies of Genital Tract

SAQ 1 What is cervical dysplasia?

Cervical dysplasia is intraepithelial neoplastic changes varying from mild degree at the base of cervical squamous epithelium to full thickness of the epithelial lining.

SAQ 2 How the cervical intraepithelial neoplasias (CIN) are graded?

They are graded as follows:

Grade I: Mild dysplasia extending one-third from basal layer.

Grade II: Moderate dysplasia extended by two-thirds of full thickness of basal layer.

Grade III: Severe dysplasia covering *in situ* covering full epithelial thickness.

SAQ 3 What are the significances of cervical dysplasia?

It may persist for several years, or small lesion may retrogress or may coexist with carcinoma in situ or invasive carcinoma.

SAQ 4 How to manage cervical dysplasia?

Repeated cytology and histological diagnoses are made by cytology, biopsy or colposcopy. In young electrocauterization or conization or cryosurgery or laser therapy. Parsistant cervical dysplasia in elderly women with completed family treated by hysterectomy.

SAQ 5 What is carcinoma *in situ*?

When the carcinoma of cervix involves the full thickness of epithelium without stromal invasion.

SAQ 6 Define carcinoma of cervix.

It is the malignant growth from epithelium of cervix invading basement membrane.

SAQ 7 What are the causes of Ca cervix?

Coitus

Sperm's nucleic acid.

Social

More in poors, Negroes.
In married or married before 20 years, multiple partners, multiparity, first sexual act before 20 yrs, prostitutes.

Infections

Syphilis, herpes II.

SAQ 8 What are the different histologic types of Ca cervix?

It may be squamous cell carcinoma mainly or adenocarcinoma.

SAQ 9 How the Ca cervix spreads?

It spreads by:

- Directly
- Lymphatics
- Blood.

SAQ 10 Mention the Border's histological grouping of Ca cervix.

Border in 1926 grouped Ca cervix histologically as follows:

(i) Grade. I: 25% undifferentiated cells
(ii) Grade II: 25–50% undifferentiated cells
(iii) Grade III: 50–75% undifferentiated cells
(iv) Grade IV: 75–100% undifferentiated cells most malignant. Most of the Ca cervix contain all grades of malignancies.

LAQ 11 Stage the Ca cervix clinically.

Stage 0

Preinvasive. Not detectable clinically.

Stage I

- **Stage I (a)**: Early stromal invasion. Undiagnosed clinically.
- **Stage I (b)**: Diagnosed clinically.

Stage II

Extends beyond cervix but not pelvic wall.

Stage III

Extends pelvic wall lower one-third of vagina.

Stage IV

Extends beyond pelvis involves bladder, rectum

SAQ 12 What do you mean by early Ca cervix and microinvasive Ca cervix?

These early stage invasive Ca cervix can be diagnosed microscopically only and there is no clinical visible lesions.

SAQ 13 How to take cervical biopsy?

It is taken by:

- Wedge biopsy
- Multiple quadrant biopsy and
- Conization

SAQ 14 What is Schiller's iodine test?

Iodine solution (prepared by I_2 1 gm; KI 2 gm and water 300 ml) applied over cervix and vault. The cancerous epithelium without glycogen is stainless and normal epithelium with glycogen stains mohogany brown. Cervical erosion, decubitus ulcer atrophied epithelium and premalignant neoplastic lesions are also Schiller's positive, i.e. unstained.

SAQ 15 Mention the important differential diagnosis of Ca cervix.

- Cervical erosion
- Mucous polyp
- Tubercular ulcer
- Syphilitic sore

LAQ 16 What are the clinical features of Ca cervix?

Married, parous rarely virgins or nulliparous in age group of 40–60 years with.

Symptoms

- Pain
- Cachexia
- Irregular bleeding
- Discharge

Signs

Speculum examination.
Papillary growth which is friable with indurated hard base. Uterus immobile in late stage P/R: Rectal wall and utero-sacral ligament indurated in advanced stage.

> Biopsy and histological examination confirms diagnosis.

SAQ 17 What are the causes of death in Ca cervix?

- Haemorrhage
- Renal failure
- Distant metastasis
- Peritonitis
- Pyometra
- PID
- RVF and VVF

SAQ 18 What is cervical stump carcinoma?

It is Ca cervix after subtotal hysterectomy may arise after 2 years of hysterectomy (true stump carcinoma) or coincident (stump carcinoma) which remains during hysterectomy.

SAQ 19 What is endometrial carcinoma?

The carcinoma which arises from endometrial epithelium and confined within uterus for long time.

LAQ 20 What are the different modes of treatment in Ca cervix?

Different types of treatment are:

Radiotherapy	**Surgery**	**Radiotherapy + Surgery**	**Chemotherapy**
All stages of Ca cervix. For stage 0, its result is equal to surgery.	[Stage I and I (a)] 1. Radical abdominal hysterectomy (Wertheim's operation). 2. Radical vaginal hysterectomy (Schauta's operation). 3. Pelvic exenteration operation (Burnschwig's operation). 4. Palliative surgery.	Stage I and II.	For advanced Ca cervix with metastatsis or pelvic recurrence after surgery with cyclophosphamide; or adriamycin or 5FU; Mtx; vincristine, mitomycin C.

LAQ 21 What are the causes of endometrial carcinoma?

- Familial tendency
- Virginity
- Nulliparity
- Late menopause
- Polyp

- Fibroid uterus
- Granulosa cell tumour
- Thecoma of ovary
- Postmesopausal oestrogen therapy
- Stein-Leventhal syndrome
- Radiation, menopause, etc. are different causes incriminated for endometrial carcinoma.

SAQ 22 What are the different modes of spread of endometrial carcinoma?

It is slow growing but may spread by:
(i) Direct spread
(ii) Lymphatic spread
(iii) Blood spread

SAQ 23 What are the different microscopic appearances of endometrial carcinoma?

Following microscopic varieties are observed for endometrial carcinoma.

- Adenocarcinoma in situ
- Adenoma malignum
- Adenocarcinoma
- Solid alveolar type
- Adenocanthoma
- Primary squamous carcinoma

LAQ 24 Stage endometrial carcinoma.

Stage 0
Carcinoma in situ.

Stage I
Confined to uterus

- I (a)
  Uterine cavity-8 cm.
- I (b)
  Uterine cavity more than 8 cm.

Stage II
Involves corpus and cervix.

Stage III
Spreaded not beyond pelvis.

Stage IV
Spreaded to extrapelvis and bladder and rectum

HISTOLOGICALLY

G1
Highly differentiated adenomatous carcinoma

G2
Differentiated adenomatous carcinoma

G3
Undifferentiated carcinoma

SAQ 25 How the endometrial carcinoma presents?

Generally occurs after menopause presents with

Symptoms

- Pain
- White discharge
- Irregular postmenopausal or intermenstrual bleeding.

Signs

- Anaemia
- Emaciation
- Enlarged abdominal inguinal gland
- Uterus is either atrophic normal or bulky.
- Cervix healthy
- Oozing of blood.
- P/R: NAD.

SAQ 26 What are the different methods of diagnosing endometrial carcinoma?

- Endometrial curettage and histology
- Vaginal pool cytological smear
- Endometrial lavage cytology
- Suction curettage
- Hysteroscopy may be helpful.

SAQ 27 How to treat endometrial carcinoma?

- Total abdominal hysterectomy with bilateral salpingo-oophorectomy.
- For Ca endometrium and endocervix: (a) Wertheim operation, (b) radiotherapy (internal and external irradiation).
- Poor risk for surgery – radiation.
- Drug therapy: Heavy and prolonged dose of progesterone. Cytotoxic drugs (methotrexate and 5FU, endoxan).

SAQ 28 What is uterine sarcoma?

The malignant tumour arising from: Muscle or vessel or fibromyoma may occur at any age infancy to childhood. It is treated surgically (total hysterectomy with bilateral salpingo-oophorectomy), chemotherapy for advanced cases with metastasis.

SAQ 29 What are the different types of carcinoma of fallopian tube?

It may be: (i) primary or (ii) from secondary deposit from uterus or ovary.

SAQ 30 What are the different types of carcinoma of vagina?

It may be: (i) primary or (ii) secondary from cervix, endometrium, ovary, rectum, choriocarcinoma or from urinary bladder.

SAQ 31 What is the treatment of carcinoma of vagina?

Surgery (Wertheim operation, vaginal radical hysterectomy) or radiotherapy.

SAQ 32 What are the different causes of leukoplakia?

These are white patches on vulva due to chronic irritation or deficiency (of B_{12}, folic acid) may be predisposed by kraurosis or lichen sclerosus.

SAQ 33 What is kraurosis?

Atrophic condition of vulva, labia minora introitus, clitoris, external urinary meatus, vestibule, frenulum but not perineum or genitocrural is called kraurosis.

SAQ 34 What is lichen sclerosis at atrophicus?

Atrophic scleroderma affecting vulva, genitocrural fold, thigh and other parts of body, starts as white papules on vulva. There is no pruritus.

LAQ 35 What are the different types of carcinoma of vulva?

Primary

- Squamous cell
- Melanoma
- Rodent ulcer

Secondary

- Cervical or endometrial carcinoma
- Choriocarcinoma
- Vaginal carcinoma

LAQ 36 What are the different causes of chronic pyometra?

The chronic retention of pus in uterine cavity called chronic pyometra occurs in the following conditions:

(i) Senile endometritis
(ii) Submucous fibroid
(iii) Radiation of uterine carcinoma
(iv) IUCD
(v) Cauterisation of cervix
(vi) Endometrial carcinoma
(vii) Endocervical carcinoma

35 Ovarian Tumours/ Radiotherapy/Chemotherapy

LAQ 1 Classify ovarian tumours.

OVARIAN TUMOUR

Common epithelial tumour

(A) Serous tumour
- Cystadenoma
- Adenocarcinoma
- Papilloma

(B) Mucinous tumours
(C) Endometroid tumour
(D) Undifferentiated carcinoma
(E) Brenner's tumour
(F) Clear cell carcinoma

Gonadal sex cord stromal tumour

(A) Granulosa theca cell tumour
(B) Fibroma sarcoma
(C) Androblastoma
(D) Gyandroblastoma

Germ cell tumour

(A) Dysgerminoma
(B) Teratoma
(C) Gonadoblastoma
(D) Choriocarcinoma
(E) Embryonal carcinoma
(F) Endodermal sinus tumour

Secondary metastasis

- Krukenberg's tumour

Tumour like condition

- Luteal cyst
- Polycystic ovary

SAQ 2 What is Brenner's tumour?

This benign fibroma consisting of islands of epithelial cell nest in fibrons stroma called Walthard bodies.

SAQ 3 What is Krukenberg's tumour?

It is secondary metastatic tumour of the ovaries arising from pylorus of stomach, spread by transperitoneal spill, or retroperitoneal lymphatic permeation or by bloodstream.

SAQ 4 What different complications may arise of ovarian tumour?

Important complications of ovarian tumours are:
- Torsion
- Adhesion
- Infection
- Rupture
- Pseudomyxoma peritonei
- Ascitis
- Malignancy

LAQ 5 How the ovarian carcinoma are staged?

Stages of ovarian cancer

Stage-I

Limited to ovaries Stage-I is subgrouped into 1(a), 1(b), 1(c).

Stage-II

One ovary involved with pelvic extension subgrouped to II and II(a)

Stage-III

Involves both ovaries with peritoneal metastasis

Stage-IV

Distant metastasis.

SAQ 6 What are the different modes of treatment of ovarian tumour?

Depending upon stage and type, the different modes of treatment are:

- Surgery
- Chemotherapy and
- Radiotherapy or their combinations.

SAQ 7 Name a masculizing ovarian tumour.

Sertoli-Leydig cell tumour (also called andro- or arrhenoblastoma)

SAQ 8 What is dermoid cyst of ovary?

It is benign cystic nature, teratoma, generally unilateral containing sebaceous material, tuff of hair, teeth of ectodermal origin.

SAQ 9 What is struma ovari?

These teratomas of ovary are spongy, solid, grayish brown contents thyroid tissues and may produce thyrotoxicosis.

SAQ 10 Name some broad ligament tumours and cysts.

Broad ligament cysts

Fimbrial cyst
Paraovarian cyst
Pseudobroad ligament cyst

Broad ligament tumours

Fibroma
Fibromyoma
Lipoma.

SAQ 11 Name the conditions where radiotherapy has scope in gynaecology.

The indications of radiotherapy in gynaecology can be grouped as follows:

Malignant conditions

(i) Ca cervix
(ii) Ca uterine body
(iii) Sarcoma of uterus (postoperatively)
(iv) Carcinoma of vagina
(v) Ca vulva
(vi) Malignant ascitis
(vii) Malignant ovarian tumour

Non-malignant conditions

(i) Pelvic endometriosis
(ii) DUB
(iii) Some cases of fibroid
(iv) To produce menopause

SAQ 12 Name the different gynaecological malignant conditions where chemotherapy is used.

(i) Choriocarcinoma (methotrexate, actinomycin D).
(ii) Ovarian carcinoma (chlorambucil, thiotepa, endoxan, alkeran, 5FU; actinomycin-D; mustine).
(iii) Tubal adenocarcinoma (alkeran, progesterone).
(iv) Pelvic sarcoma (radio + chemotherapy).
(v) Epidermoid carcinoma: Poor responder to chemotherapy.

SAQ 13 Name some retroperitoneal tumours.

RETROPERITONEAL TUMOURS

Benign

- Lipoma
- Fibroma
- Ganglioma

Malignant

Primary

- Lymphosarcoma
- Leiomyosarcoma
- Anaplastic carcinoma

Secondary

From pelvis and ovary

Backache, Pruritus Vulvae; Leukorrhoea

36

SAQ 1 What is pruritus vulvae?

Itching of vulva and surrounding area due to leukorrhoea, leukoplakia, kraurosis, uncleanness, strong soap, parasites, eczema and other dermatological conditions. Anaemia, vitamin A; B deficiency; diabetes, idiopathic, psychoneurosis, etc.

LAQ 2 What are causes of low backache in female?

The different causes can be grouped as follows:

Non-gynaecological causes

- **Orthopaedic causes**
  - Sacroiliac strain
  - Muscular and ligamentary strain
  - Arthritis
  - Sacralization of lumbar vertebrae
  - Lumbago
  - Coccygodynia
- **Non-orthopaedic causes**
  - Renal and rectal causes

Gynaecological causes

- Prolapse
- Retroversion
- TO mass
- Endometritis
- Premenstrual
- Parametritis

SAQ 3 What is leukorrhoea?

Any discharge apart from blood, stool, urine per vagina may be due to:

(i) Physiological – during early pregnancy, ovulation, sexual excitement.

(ii) Pathological – vulvovaginitis; foreign body in vagina, trichomoniosis, gonorrhoea, bartholinitis, cervical erosion, uterine polyp, decubitus ulcer, prolapse, fibroid, uterine cancer, prolapse, pessary, endometritis, pyometra, etc.

SAQ 4 What is Behçet's syndrome?

Vulval ulcer, conjunctivitis, keratitis, which appear in relation to particular phase of menstruation. The etiology is not known.

SAQ 5 What is Esthiomene?

Chronic vulval ulcer with associated hypertrophy.

Paediatric and Geriatric Gynaecology

37

LAQ 1 What are the different causes of precocious puberty?

True precocious puberty

- Constitutional
- Intracranial lesion
- Endocranial
- Albright's syndrome

Pseudo-precocious puberty

- Granulosa cell tumour
- Thecoma
- Teratoma
- Oestrogen
- Adrenocortical neoplasm
- Androgen ingestion
- End organ sensitivity producing thelarche and puberche

LAQ 2 Mention some geriatric gynaecological problems.

- Menopausal syndrome
- Delayed menopause
- Pruritus vulvae
- Senile vaginitis
- Ca cervix
- Ovarian tumour
- Ca fallopian tube
- Prolapse of genitalia
- Bleeding P/R
- Atonic constipation
- Dysuria
- Rectal prolapse, etc.

38 Oestrogen and Progesterone Hormone Therapy

SAQ 1 What are the sources of oestrogens?

Oestrogen induces oestrous in animals. In human being, oestradiol, secreted by ovary, is the major source of it. It is also synthesized by graafian follicles, corpus luteum and placenta.

SAQ 2 How does oestrogen act?

It binds to cytoplasmic receptors in target cells to regulate protein synthesis via nucleus.

SAQ 3 Name some oestrogen preparations.

Steroidal

- Ethinyloestradiol
- Mestranol
- Tibolone

Non-steroidal

- Diethylstilbestrol (orally).
- Hexesterol and divestrol (topically).

LAQ 4 Mention some therapeutic uses of oestrogen.

- Senile vaginitis
- Hormone replacement therapy
- Delayed puberty in girls
- Dysmenorrhoea
- Acne
- Hirsutism
- DUB
- Suppression of lactation
- Ca prostate
- OCP

SAQ 5 What is transdermal oestradiol (oestradiol TTS)?

These are used to treat menopausal syndrome available in sizes 5,10, 20 cm^2 delivering 0, 0.25 mg; 0.05 mg and 0.1 mg in 24 hours.

SAQ 6 What are the function of progesterone and what is its mechanism of action?

In broad sense, it converts, oestrogen primed endometrium to secretory phase to maintain pregnancy. It acts on specific receptors in target cells (female genital tract, breast, CNS and pituitary), translocated to nucleus producing RNA transcription to regulate protein synthesis.

LAQ 7 What are the therapeutic uses of progesterone?

- Contraceptive
- Hormone replacement in postmenopausal women
- DUB
- Endometriosis
- Premenstrual tension
- Threatened abortion and habitual abortion
- Metastatic endometrial carcinoma as palliative treatment

SAQ 8 What is mifepristone?

It is competitive antiprogesterone and antiglucocorticoid given in follicular phase acts as partial agonist of progesterone used for:

- Termination of pregnancy
- Contragestational
- Inoperable Cushing's syndrome
- To induce labour
- Fibroid of uterus

SAQ 9 Name some progesterone preparations.

- Dihydrogesterone
- Megestrol
- Ethisterone
- Dimethisterone
- Norethisterone
- Norethynodral
- Lynosterol
- Norgesteral

LAQ 10 What are the important adverse effects of oestrogen and progesterone?

Adverse effects of oestrogen	Adverse effects of progesterone
Suppresses libido and gynecomastia in male when given for Ca prostate; Early fusion of epiphysis; increases incidences of vaginal and cervical carcinoma; in postmenopausal women chances of gallstone, hepatoma, migraine and endometriosis are worsened.	Headache, breast engorgement, rise of body temperature, amenorrhoea or irregular bleeding, lower HDL, blood sugar may rise masculinization of foetus with congenital anomalies.

39 Operations in Gynaecology

LAQ 1 What is hysterectomy? What are its types?

Removal of uterus by operation:

By route

- Abdominal
- Vaginal

Types

I Total	II Subtotal	III* Panhysterectomy	IV* Radical hysterectomy
Entire uterus	Only corpus	Total + bilateral salpingo-oophorectomy.	Total + bilateral salpingo-oophorectomy + Removal of parametrium + upper vagina + pelvic

SAQ 2 What are the contraindications of vaginal hysterectomy?

- PID
- Large uterus
- Endometriosis
- Cervical hypertrophy
- Ovarian tumour
- Pelvic irradiated
- Post-laparotomy
- Normal uterus without descent.

SAQ 3 What is D/C operation?

In this operation, cervix is dilated and uterine cavity is curetted.

* For neoplastic conditions

LAQ 4 What are the indications of hysterectomy?

Congenital
- Rudimentary horn

Acquired

- **Traumatic**: Perforation
- **Inflammatory**: PID, Haematocele
- **Neoplastic**: Fibroma, Endometriosis
- **Miscellaneous**:
  - DUB
  - Prolapse

LAQ 5 What are the important complications of hysterectomy?

Operative
- Injury to bladder or rectum
- Haemorrhage
- Anaesthetic hazard

Postoperative
- Shock
- Infection
- Vomiting
- Paralytic ileus
- Bronchopneumonia
- Wound complications
- Vault prolapse
- Thrombosis

Remote
- Menopausal syndrome
- Arthralgia
- Coronary disease

LAQ 6 What are the indications of D/C operation?

Indications for D/C
- Dysmenorrhoea
- DUB
- Polyp
- Oligomenorrhoea
- Dysmenorrhoea (TB)
- Infertility
- Endometrial carcinoma
- Choriocarcinoma.

Indications of only dilatation
- Spasmodic dysmenorrhoea
- Insufflation for tubal patency
- Cervical amputation
- Radium insertion
- Cautery
- Draining pyometra
- Cervical stenosis

Indications of only curettage
- For endometrial biopsy.

SAQ 7 What complications may arise out of D/C operation?

Following complications may arise out of D/C operations:

- Injury of cervix and bleeding
- Uterine perforation
- Laparotomy
- Bowel injury
- Infection
- Synechia
- Secondary amenorrhoea